Sleep and Society

"This   or
socio   d'
socio   however,   ns
lend   al
result   sleep.
Willi

                                                                  Exeter, UK

We s   e of these
great   a daily or
night   historically
varia   and other
resea   the social
dimer

Sleep   through
this l   changing
theor   a-cultural
varia   lifeworld,
sleep   of sleep,
and t

Writt   nd many
timely, topical and original insights, *Sleep and Society* will appeal to a truly inter-
disciplinary audience, including students and researchers within the social sciences
and humanities, sleep scientists, and other professionals, practitioners and policy
makers with an interest in sleep-related matters.

Simon J. Williams is Reader in Sociology at the University of Warwick. He has published widely within the sociology of health, the sociology of the body, and the sociology of emotions. He is currently involved in a range of sleep-related research
projects and is co-organiser of the new Economic and Social Research Council
(ESRC) seminar series on 'Sleep and Society'.

Sleep and Society

Sociological ventures into the (un)known . . .

Simon J. Williams

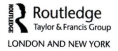
Routledge
Taylor & Francis Group

LONDON AND NEW YORK

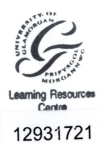
First published in 2005 by Routledge
2 Park Square, Milton Park, Abingdon,
Oxfordshire, OX14 4RN
Tel: +44 020 7017 6000
Fax: +44 020 7017 6699

Simultaneously published in the USA and Canada
by Taylor & Francis Inc
270 Madison Ave, New York, NY 10016

Routledge is an imprint of the Taylor & Francis Group

© 2005 Simon J. Williams

Typeset in Sabon by J&L Composition, Filey, North Yorkshire
Printed and bound in Great Britain by TJ International Ltd,
Padstow, Cornwall

Every effort has been made to ensure that the advice and information in this book are true and accurate at the time of going to
press. However, neither the publisher nor the authors can accept
any legal responsibility or liability for any errors or omissions
that may be made. In the case of drug administration, any medical
procedure or the use of technical equipment mentioned within
this book, you are strongly advised to consult the manufacturer's
guidelines.

British Library Cataloguing in Publication Data
A catalogue record for this book is available from the British
Library

Library of Congress Cataloging in Publication Data
A catalog record has been requested

ISBN 0–415–35418–8 (hbk)
ISBN 0–415–35419–6 (pbk)

To Fish and Chips and a life well-slept

Contents

Acknowledgements   viii

Preface   x

Introduction   1

1 Changing theories and explanations of sleep:
   from ancient to modern times   9

2 Sleep through the centuries: historical patterns
   and practices   37

3 Sleep, embodiment and the lifeworld (*Lebenswelt*)   67

4 The social patterning and social organisation of sleep:
   inequalities, institutions and injustices   101

5 Colonising/capitalising on sleep? Medicalisation
   and beyond . . .   143

Conclusions: remaining questions and the challenges ahead   169

References   173

Index   193

Acknowledgements

Thanks to the University of Warwick for granting me the sabbatical time necessary to write this book and to my colleagues in the Department of Sociology, particularly Margaret Archer, Jim Beckford, Robert Fine and Deborah Lynn Steinberg, for their encouragement and support in this venture. Frances Griffiths and Pamela Lowe in the Centre for Primary Health Care Studies have also stuck by me through thick and thin on the sleep research front: thanks to you both for your continuing support, we are getting there! Thanks also go to Christine Bradford, in the Library, for help and assistance with various literature searches, to Jonathan Reinarz for some useful historical sources, to Rob Lee for pointing me in the direction of Ballard on the horrors of continuous wakefulness and to Chris Yuill for some old Gaelic references to sleep. The Bodelian library, University of Oxford, proved an invaluable resource for which I am very grateful. Many other people also deserve mention, including: Peter Conrad, Tom Crook, Kenton Kroker, Kevin Morgan and Neil Stanley, who all in various ways shared their thoughts with me regarding the nature and status of 'sleep medicine' and the medicalisation of sleep, both past and present; Nick Crossley, for discussions about sleep, embodiment and the lifeword; Paul Higgs for our discussions of the nature and status of sleep as a sociological issue or project; Chris Shilling for the important sociological points raised in his role as discussant at the first Economic and Social Research Council (ESRC) 'Sleep and Society' seminar; Bryan Turner for insightful comments on the 'socially attentive sleeper' and for his general support and encouragement in respect of this (post)dormative project; Charles Leadbeater for our discussion and debate on sleep in the 24/7 society; and Sara Arber and colleagues at the University of Surrey for their collaborative efforts in helping take forward our new ESRC 'Sleep and Society' seminar series – something, in conjunction with this book, which should I hope put sleep firmly on the sociological research agenda. Thanks too, of course, go to Karen Bowler and all at Routledge for ensuring the smooth and safe passage of this book through the production process. Last but certainly not least, thanks to Ruth Charity who has not simply enthused about the book from start to finish but has carefully read and commented on every page. The book, I hope, does everyone justice. The errors, of course, are mine and mine alone.

Preface

This book has been a *pleasure* and a *pain* to write: a pleasure, because sleep is such a rich and fascinating topic and because most of the research and writing was done whilst I was on sabbatical; a pain because my sleep life has doubtless suffered (the more I researched sleep the less sleep I seemed to get, initially at least) and because there is a dearth of literature of the kind I wished or hoped for bearing *directly* on the social let alone the *sociological* dimensions of sleep. I have therefore, faced with this latter conundrum, relied heavily and unashamedly on those precious few sources that speak directly to the themes of this book, whilst simultaneously casting the net far and wide for other *indirect, hidden,* or *oblique* references of this kind: a two-fold strategy of investigative work, in effect, successful or not. Everybody however seems to have a story to tell about sleep, or lack of it, which underlined my conviction that this was a book worth writing and that sleep was indeed a legitimate topic of sociological investigation. Some, no doubt, in sociology and beyond, will wish to quibble. Nonetheless, to the extent that this book provides a catalyst for subsequent sociological work in this 'dormant' domain it will indeed have served its purpose. On that, of course, I leave you the reader to judge. . .

Simon J. Williams
May 2005

Introduction

Some must watch while some must sleep
(Shakespeare, *Hamlet*, Act III, Scene II)

This is a book about *Sleep and Society*, an invitation to enter a largely uncharted terrain, sociologically speaking at least, and to see things differently in doing so. It is a book about socially, culturally and historically variable matters such as *how* we sleep, *when* we sleep, *where* we sleep and with *whom* we sleep, including the *meanings, methods, motives* and *management* of sleep or sleep*ing* in everyday/every night life (cf. Taylor 1993). It is also a book about changing attitudes, ideas, beliefs, explanations and understandings of sleep in lay, popular and professional culture, both past and present.

Sleep is a crucial if not vital part of our lives, a basic human *right* in fact, acknowledged or not. Approximately a third of our lives is taken up with this weird and wonderful pursuit or pastime, itself a source of pleasure or pain depending on your success as a sleeper. We are sleeping as well as waking beings, with a rich dream life to boot. Sleep, moreover, rightly or wrongly, is strongly associated in words and deeds with issues of time, wealth, wisdom and moral virtue. Proverbs and aphorisms abound to this effect: 'Early to bed and early to rise makes man healthy, wealthy and wise', for instance, is one among many such terms of reference. Literature is full of references to the pleasures and pains of sleep, from Shakespeare to Proust, Dickens to de la Mare, Coleridge to Cervantes. To study sleep, however, or even to entertain the possibility of doing so, opens up a number of sociological problems, puzzles or paradoxes. Why, for example, if sleep is so critical or central to our lives, has it been so neglected as a topic of serious sustained sociological reflection or investigation? Why is it only now that sociologists are beginning (emphasis on beginning) to turn their attention to this neglected issue? What does a sociological approach to sleep involve or entail, and where precisely does it begin and end? Is a sociological approach to sleep possible given the predominant waking concerns of the discipline? Is there a tension or contradiction, in the current (global) era, between the seemingly 'incessant' demands of the 24/7 waking world and our continuing need to sleep? Is 'too much' or 'too little' sleep, whatever that might mean, a 'problem' or 'threat' to society? How does this square, moreover, with current debates on risk society, the changing pace or tempo of social life, or with growing media interest in sleep-related matters – from tips on how to sleep well, to infra red camera footage of people's strange behaviour whilst asleep, and from the recent UK Channel 4 'Shattered' sleep deprivation contest, to front-page coverage of David Beckham's sleep life in the name of art[1]?

These are some of the questions and issues that this book seeks to address if not answer in the chapters that follow. The prime focus or emphasis, it should be stressed, is *sociological*, although I draw on a wide range of sources in pursuit of these sociological themes and issues; a recasting or translation, in effect, or perhaps more uncharitably a pillaging and plundering, of much past and present work along these lines. This includes a close re-reading of many classic and contemporary sources, in sociology and beyond, with sleep in mind. There is, as we shall see, much implicit if not explicit material here already for us to mine for sociological insights. Sleep, moreover, is not simply a rich and fascinating sociological topic in its own right, it also provides a new way or means of approaching other well established sociological research topics and agendas: another lens or window, in effect, onto the social world of everyday/every night life.

So what then of this alleged past sociological neglect? And why this newly emerging interest in sleep?

Sociology and sleep: an odd couple or intimate bedfellows?

When I first became interested in sleep back in 1998, the first thing that struck me was the paucity of sociological literature bearing directly on this topic. The more I thought about sleep, the more sociologically important it became, and the more odd it seemed that sociologists had overlooked or neglected it as a serious topic of investigation. Yes, there had been some important and insightful ventures or forays in this direction over the years, including notable papers by Aubert and White (1959a,b), Schwartz (1970) and more recently Taylor (1993) on the sociological dimensions of sleep, but the general impression held good that sleep, by and large, was something of a blind spot as far as sociologists were concerned.

The field, instead, appeared to be dominated by the work of sleep science in its manifold guises, together with other psychological and philosophical insights into sleep, dreams and dreaming, and psychoanalytic interpretations of the latter as the 'royal road', in Freud's famous terms, 'to the unconscious'. Sociologists, however, were far from the odd ones out here.

Anthropologists and historians too, it seemed, had similarly neglected sleep. The study of the social life it seemed, both past and present, stopped dead in its tracks when people went to bed, or perhaps more correctly 'fell asleep': the two are far from synonymous of course.

These impressions were confirmed and compounded on numerous occasions when I floated the possibilities of a sociology of sleep, or something similar. 'A sociology of sleep?', people would say, 'You must be joking, whatever next!' A colleague, in fact, once confessed to me that he thought I must have submitted a spoof paper on reading the title 'towards a sociology of sleep' in the conference programme. Alternatively, people would ask if I had a sleep disorder (I do not by the way, to the best of my knowledge) or assumed that it must be dreams or dreaming I was interested in. Dreaming, for understandable reasons perhaps, appears to have received the lion's share of attention in the history of humankind. Sleep of course is a necessary condition for dreaming, but it is sleep, in the main, that I am interested in as a sociological research topic or problematic, without in any way discounting the social or sociological significance of dreams or the dreamer.

These responses and reactions are themselves, however, sociologically interesting; revealing much about the past/present preferences or prejudices of our own discipline, and its predominant waking concerns, which effectively banish, discard or dismiss sleep (given the loss of waking consciousness involved) as an 'a-social' or 'non-social', if not downright 'anti-social', event or experience and an involuntary form of 'in-action' (cf. Taylor 1993), thereby leaving it to the tender mercies of disciplines such as biology, physiology, psychology or what is now collectively known as sleep science and/or sleep medicine. It may reasonably be objected that to venture into this terrain surely risks the charge of sociological imperialism given these other vested disciplinary interests in this dormant domain.

Further reflection, nonetheless, reveals the limits of any such reading, response or riposte. Sleep, as we shall see, is far from sociologically unimportant or uninteresting; no mere biological 'given' or a-social event, that is to say, it is, instead, a complex (learned) behaviour or practice that displays a high degree of *socio-cultural plasticity* or *variability*. Sleep, to put it more formally or schematically, is *irreducible* to any one domain or discourse, arising or *emerging* through the interplay of biological and psychological processes, environmental and structural circumstances (qua facilitators and constraints), and socio-cultural forms of elaboration, conceived in temporally, spatially, contextually bounded and embodied terms. Relations between the sleeping and waking world, moreover, are themselves complex and mutually reinforcing.

To understand sleep or sleeping, as this suggests, we need to understand a good deal about people's social lives, social roles and social relationships. Attention to people's sleep, reciprocally, sheds important light on their social lives, social roles and social relationships. Far from being mere 'isolated' behaviour or 'time out', sleep only makes sense when placed in the context of people's everyday/night lives, including the social networks within which it is embodied and embedded (cf. Crossley 2004). Sleep, moreover, from the viewpoint of society, is far too important to be left to mere biological 'whim' or 'dictate'. All societies, in one way or another, are confronted with the 'problem' of how to organise or institutionalise the sleeping as well as the waking life of their members: hence the questions posed above of the *how*, *when*, *where* and *with whom* variety. On the one hand, sleep may pose a significant 'challenge', 'problem' or 'threat' to society, particularly if 'too many' people sleep for 'too long' – itself of course a socially and culturally defined matter. On the other hand, the same may very well be said of 'too little' sleep on the part of 'too many'. Sleep, in this respect, is a socially regulated/controlled, socially organised/institutionalised state or practice, which, without wishing to sound too functionalist, is crucial (in proper proportion or measure) to society and the health and well being of each and every one of us, acknowledged or not. In short, 'Some must sleep', to place the emphasis somewhat differently to Shakespeare, 'while some must watch'.

Herein lie the beginnings or bare bones then of an answer as to why sociologists should perhaps consider or reconsider sleep as a legitimate topic worthy of their attention. Unless and until sleep is addressed, a third of our life remains missing from the sociological landscape, or to put it slightly differently, only two thirds of the sociological job is done. The same indeed may well be said of recent attempts to bring the body (back) in to sociology, which likewise remain incomplete without adequate attention to these 'dormant' or perhaps not so dormant matters. As for whether this need to (re)consider sleep also involves or entails a reconceptualisation, recovery or reclaiming of sleep in one way or another, these are issues that run through the book as a whole and ones we shall return to and fully spell out in the conclusion.

What is clear up front, as this preliminary discussion suggests, is that the (sociological) analysis or exploration of sleep and society may operate on at least three interrelated levels – see Table 1 below. The first *individual/(non)experiential* level, concerns phenomenological issues to do with what one might provisionally term the dormant, dreaming or drowsy body, including (non)experiential matters such as falling or being asleep, nonconscious activities or events such as snoring, sleep walking, sleep talking and the like, subjective feelings of sleepiness and related issues to do with the relationships between sleep and (alert) wakefulness. Sleep, as this suggests, is a *liminal* (betwixt and between) state that exists somewhere in the borderlands between consciousness and unconsciousness, including both the voluntary and the involuntary, the purposive and the non-purposive, the personal and the impersonal, the biological and the social, the universal and

Table 1 Sleep and Society: levels of analysis

Level	Problem	Key concept(s)	Perspective(s) (Examples)
Individual/ (non)experiential	Falling/being asleep, (un/non) consciousness, snoring, sleep walking/talking etc., sleepiness	Dormant/dreaming/ drowsy body; 'depth disappearance'/ (recessive) embodiment	Phenomenology
Social/ interactional	Meanings, methods, motives, management	'Doing'/negotiating sleep*ing*; sleep role, rituals; gender; life course	Interactionism, sociology of ED/NL; sociology of norms, roles, deviance; feminism(s)
Societal/ institutional	Order/organisation, power, structure, spatialisation, surveillance	Civilizing sleep disciplining/ regulating sleep; public/private; social patterning of sleep	Elias, Foucault, medicalisation, political economy . . .

the specific. I cannot, for example, directly audit my own sleep qua sleeper, though I can infer a good deal about its nature, quantity and quality upon waking. Nor can I simply will myself to sleep, try as I might, though I can take a series of (reflexive) steps or measures to encourage or discourage it (cf. Leder 1990; Crossley 2004). These latter (reflexive) elements or dimensions of sleep in turn key into the second *social/interactional* level, which Taylor (1993) has usefully termed the sociological 'doing' of sleep or to be more precise the doing of sleep*ing* – the (gendered) meanings, methods, motives and management of sleeping, that is to say, and the 'negotiation' of sleeping in everyday/every night life. Relevant sociological perspectives here, as this suggests, include interactionist theory in its various guises and the sociology of norms, roles and deviance, together with other feminist/gender and life course perspectives and approaches to sleep and sleeping. The third *societal/institutional* level of analysis brings into focus or play broader sociological issues to do with the social patterning, scheduling, spatialisation and organisation of sleep across the public/private divide, and related questions to do with risk, regulation, medicalisation and surveillance. Eliasian, Foucauldian and political economy perspectives, for instance, are among a range of options available here, each yielding their own important insights when turned to sleep-related matters. These levels of analysis, to repeat, are far from mutually exclusive. Nor are they exhaustive: a beginning rather than an end point, one might say.

How then are these initial insights carried forward or cashed out in the book?

Sleep and society: an outline

The first chapter of this book takes a step back, so to speak, from these introductory sociological remarks, in order to examine in a preliminary fashion the prior question: what is sleep (for)? Doing so, as we shall see, takes us on a rich and fascinating journey through changing theories, ideas and explanations of sleep and dreams, including philosophical, scientific and literary sources, from pre-modern times to the present day. This itself, however, gives rise to yet another paradox concerning sleep: for all this effort over the centuries, we are still no further forward in understanding what sleep is *for*. A working definition of sleep, nonetheless, is tentatively put forward at the end of the chapter as a way of drawing these diverse themes and issues together.

The next chapter (Chapter 2) moves us from these changing theories and explanations of sleep through the ages to changing patterns and practices of sleep across the centuries. We return to Elias's work on the civilizing process, for example, for insights into the privatisation or sequestration of sleep, alongside Foucauldian and Weberian insights on the disciplined/docile if not dormant body. These insights, in turn, are augmented through further historical work on sleep in pre-industrial times, the spatialisation of 'dormant' bodies in Victorian England, including the problems of over-crowding, and a brief supplementary history of the bed.

Chapter 3 moves us more squarely on to questions of embodiment, and the (reflexive) links this provides to the doing and negotiation of sleep or sleeping in everyday/every night life. Key themes here include a phenomenological exploration of falling asleep and being asleep, the rights and duties of the 'sleep role', the gendered doing and negotiation of sleeping across the life course, the relationship between sleep, sexuality and intimacy, and, finally, the literal and metaphorical links between sleep and death.

From here the analysis proceeds in Chapter 4 to an exploration of the social and cultural patterning of sleep, in which issues of inequality, institutions and injustices loom large. From evidence and debates as to whether or not we are all (chronically) sleep deprived to sleeping arrangements in day-care centres, hospitals, prisons and nursing homes, and from cultures of sleep around the globe to the trials and tribulations of sleeping on/off the job, to say nothing of the merits of workplace naps and the drive for ever more efficient sleep, the issues addressed here are many and varied. This, in turn, is buttressed towards the end of the chapter with some further reflections on sleep as a basic human right and resource, and the 'uses' and 'abuses' or 'rights' and 'wrongs' of sleep, both past and present.

Chapter 5 takes us from these important issues to a related series of debates on the fate of sleep in contemporary times, with particular reference to issues of medicalisation and commercialisation. The question of whether or not sleep is the latest chapter or yet another unwritten chapter in the medicalisation story is discussed and debated, together with an exploration of the many different ways in which sleep is being 'colonized' or 'capitalised' on in late/postmodernity, including the manufacture and marketing of a host of sleep-related 'goods', products and services for the tired or weary consumer to purchase and consume for that (elusive) sound or silent (night's) sleep.

A brief conclusion pays particular reference to remaining questions and the challenges ahead. Sleep, it is concluded, is not simply a rich and fascinating sociological topic in its own right, but a new way of seeing and configuring existing sociological research agendas. Seen in this light, we have little to lose and much to gain from opening our eyes and waking up to the *sociological significance of sleep*.

Notes

1 The reference here is to media reportage of Sam Taylor Wood's 67-minute long film loop of Beckham asleep at the National Portrait Gallery, London.

Chapter 1

Changing theories and explanations of sleep: from ancient to modern times

Introduction

Sleep has always been one of those great mysteries of life, something we all do but no less mysterious for that. In this chapter I take a preliminary look at the nature and status of sleep, and at attempts to unravel its causes, complexities and mysteries, with particular reference to some of the main philosophical, scientific and literary sources and contributions to this debate through the ages, from ancient to modern times: a history of changing ideas, theories and explanations of sleep, or the social construction of sleep if you like, including past and present discourses and debates on the pains if not the pathologies of sleep and the weird and wonderful world of dreams and dreaming, albeit as subsidiary themes. The chapter, in this respect, provides a first stab at the nature and status of the phenomenon under investigation and a backdrop to some of the other more sociological themes and issues that follow.

What then do we 'know' about the nature and status of sleep, and how have these ideas, theories and explanations changed or evolved over time?

Past theories and evolving ideas: from 'passive' to 'active' sleep?

Sleep has fascinated (and frustrated) people since time immemorial, with many different ideas and explanations put forward as to its nature and its causes through the ages, both Eastern and Western, 'passive' and 'active' in kind, including ancient Mesopotamian, Egyptian and Chinese beliefs and practices dating way back to 3000BC.

For our purposes, however, somewhat arbitrarily perhaps, it is to Ancient Greek thought that we first turn in search of answers to these questions. Theories and explanations of sleep were clearly and systematically articulated at this time by many great writers in the history of Western thought. Alcmaeon, for example, in the fifth century BC, has been credited with what is possibly the 'first theory of the cause of sleep', postulating that sleep occurred when the blood vessels of the brain filled with blood, with wake-fulness restored through withdrawal of blood from the brain: an early vas-cular 'congestion' theory, that is to say (Thorpy 1991: xvi). Hippocrates (460–370BC), the father of Western medicine, also speculated on the cause of sleep, believing, contra Alcmaeon, that it was due to blood going in the opposite direction, from the limbs to the inner regions or central parts of the body, where it was warmed, thereby resulting in sleep (Dannenfeldt 1986; Thorpy 1991).

Aristotle (384–322BC) contributed further to these debates through his own deliberations on sleep and dreams in *Parva Naturalia*. Sleep, Aristotle reasoned, in an early formulation of what later came be known as a 'chem-ical' theory, was due to the effects of food digestion. 'Fumes' produced through digestion, he believed, were transported in the blood vessels to the brain, which subsequently cooled and descended to the lower parts of the body, thereby taking heat away from the brain and hence inducing sleep. As he put it:

> . . . sleep is not every incapacity of the sensitive faculty. This affection arises from the evaporation of food; for that which is vaporized must be driven forward for a space, and then turn and change its course, like the tide in a narrow strait. Now in every animal the hot tends to rise; when it reaches the upper parts, it turns back and descends in a dense mass. So sleepiness mostly occurs after food, for then both liquid and solid matter are carried up in considerable bulk. As this becomes stationary it weighs one down and makes him nod; when it has shifted downwards, and by its return has driven back the hot, then sleep occurs, and the animal falls asleep.
>
> (1957: 337)

As to the question of the prophecy of dreams, Aristotle was rightly cau-tious. Most cases of the fulfilment of dreams, he reasons, are probably pure coincidence. Dreams may have medical significance, however, given that slight physical disturbances may trigger the imagination. The experiences of dreams, moreover, may modify subsequent waking conduct. There is no evidence though, Aristotle concluded, that dreams have a divine origin.

Aristotelian views, to be sure, were influential. Other theories based on 'atomism', however, were also evident in classical Roman times. Leucippus (c. 430BC), for instance, regarded sleep as a product of the partial or com-plete spinning-off of 'atoms'; a theory subsequently revived by Epicurus (c. 300BC), whose extensive writings on sleep and dreams have, sadly, been lost (Thorpy 1991).

Perhaps the next major landmark, as far as theories of sleep go, takes us through the Middle Ages and late Renaissance, where Hippocratic, Aristotelian and Galenic theories held sway (see, for example Dannenfeldt

1986), to the 'mechanistic' deliberations of René Descartes in *Treatise of Man* (1971): what Thorpy (1991: xviii) dubs a 'hydraulic model' of sleep. The brain, for Descartes, exists in two states: *waking*, in which its fibres are strong yet rapidly exhausted (due both to the fact that the spirit's source, in the blood, is used rapidly and not adequately recirculated, and that in wakefulness the admixture of blood with chyle has a 'coarsening effect'); and *sleeping*, in which its fibres are lax and its spirits gradually replenished. Exhaustion of these strong or forceful spirits in a waking person results in sleep. As this supply of spirits increases in the sleeping person, they awaken. Descartes, interestingly, resorts to a slack-sail analogy here to illustrate these processes, with dream sleep associated with general laxness, dreaming with local tension or turgor, and waking with general tension or turgor (i.e. the fully stretched sail). As Descartes puts it, in his own inimicable machine-like way:

> . . . during sleep the substance of the brain, being in repose, has leisure to be nourished and repaired, being moistened by the blood contained in the little veins and arteries that are apparent on its external surface. When, after some time, the pores, having narrowed, the spirits need be less strong to keep the brain substance quite tense (just as the wind need be less strong to inflate the ship's sails when damp than dry). And yet these spirits [in the brain] are stronger [during sleep than at other times], inasmuch as the blood producing them purified while passing and repassing several times through the heart. . ..When it follows that this machine must naturally wake itself up after it has slept for some time, just as, reciprocally, it must also go to sleep again after it has been for some time awake; for, during waking, the substance of the brain is dried out and its pores are gradually enlarged by the continual action of the spirits [Whence it also follows], that, if it [the machine] happens to eat (which hunger will incite it to do at times, if something to eat can be found), the juice of the food, on admixture with the blood, render the latter more coarse and this makes it produce fewer spirits.
>
> (1971: 110)

These views were subsequently elaborated by the famous neurologist Thomas Willis (1621–75), amongst others, whose book *The London Practices of Physick*, published in 1692, devoted considerable space to sleep-related matters. In keeping with Descartes, the animals spirits were seen to undergo rest during sleep. Some animals' spirits, however, remained 'active' in the cerebellum during sleep, in order to maintain 'control' over physiology, whilst others became intermittently 'unrestrained', resulting in dreams (Thorpy 1991: xix). The essence of sleep, Willis states:

. . . consists in this, that the corporeal soul withdrawing itself a little, and contracting the sphere of its Irradiation, in the first place renders destitute the outward part of the Brain or its cortext, and then all the outward Organs of Sense and Motion of the Emanation of the Spirits, and closes the Doors as it were; so that they being called in for refreshment sake, lye down, and indulge themselves to rest; mean while the pores and passages of the outward part of the brain being free, and void of Excursions of the Spirits afford a passage to the Nervous Liquour distilled from the Blood for new Stores of Spirits: In natural and usual sleep, these two concauses conspire and happen together as it were by some compact of Nature: viz. at the same time the Spirits recede, and that Nervous humour enters: but in nonnatural, or extraordinary Sleep, sometimes this cause, sometimes that is first: for either the Spirits being weary or called away withdraw themselves first, and afford an enterance to the Nervous humour heaped together in a readiness for it; or a plenty of Nervous humour coming to those places, and making a way by force as it were, repels the Spirits, and entering their Passages, floats them as it were.

(1692: 390)

These ideas, it seems, were still very much in evidence in the eighteenth century, albeit with further unresolved questions. Francis de Valangin, for example, in his *Treatise on Diet, or the Management of Human Life* (1768), proclaimed that sleep:

. . . is a natural Cessation of all external Perceptions, necessary for the Preservation of the animal economy. The cause of such an extraordinary State, in which external senses are thus overcome, has been the object of the Inquiries of many Philosophers. It certainly appears to proceed from Diminution or Cessation of the Influx of the animal Spirits or nervous Fluid, from the Brain into the Organs of Sense. But how this comes about, and what in reality the Impediment is that prevents the nervous Influence from the Brain into the Organs of Sensation, is a Matter not yet clearly understood. . ..

(1768: 268)

Experiments with plants may sound like something of a detour in this context, but the 'chronobiological experiments' of Jean Jacques d'ortous de Mairan in 1729 were also something of landmark as far as latter-day sleep science is concerned (Dement 2000). By placing a heliotrope plant in a darkened closet, and observing that the plant still opened its leaves during the day and closed them at night, without external time cues, the presence of circadian rhythms was first demonstrated.

Other important developments in the eighteenth century, included Albrecht von Haller's (1708–77) 'vascular' theory of sleep, based on pressure on the brain – a variant, in effect, on Alcmaeon's fifth century BC theory – which itself was expanded in the nineteenth century into a full-fledged 'congestion' theory of sleep (Thorpy 1991: xx). Perhaps most important of all, however, was Luigi Galvini's (1737–98) demonstration of the electrical activity of the nervous system, which subsequently led to the development of electrophysiology and the electroencephalograph (EEG).

The nineteenth century may be regarded as the 'age of sleep theories' (Thorpy 1991), including the flowering of 'vascular' (mechanical, anaemic, congestive), 'chemical' (humoural), 'neural' (histological) and 'behavioural' (psychological, biological) theories (see Kleitman 1963/1939 for a definitive account).

The congestive theory (i.e. pressure on the brain), for example, was the most accepted vascular theory in the first half of the nineteenth century: a theory supported by the likes of Robert MacNish, a member of the Faculty of Physicians and Surgeons of Glasgow, who wrote an influential volume on sleep and its disorders entitled *The Philosophy of Sleep* (first published in 1830 and subsequently revised and updated as a second edition in 1859). Sleep, MacNish states on the opening pages of the book of the second edition:

> ... is the intermediate state between wakefulness and death; wakefulness being regarded as the active state of all the animal intellectual functions, and death as that of their total suspension.
>
> (1859: 9)

Sleep, he continues, exists in two states: one 'complete' the other 'incomplete'. The former is said to be characterised by a 'torpor of the various organs which compose the brain, and that by the external senses and voluntary motion'. Incomplete sleep or dreaming, in contrast, is said to be the 'active' state of the one or more of the cerebral organs, while the remainder are in repose: the senses and the volition being either suspended or in action according to the circumstances of the case. Complete sleep, MacNish boldly proclaims, 'is a temporary metaphysical death, though not an organic one – the heart and lungs performing their offices with their accustomed regularity under the control of the voluntary muscles' (1859: 9).

This, Dement comments, exemplifies the overarching historical dichotomy of sleep research – 'sleep as a passive process versus sleep as an active process' (2000: 2). Studies by physiologists in the early to mid-1800s, for instance, including Luigi Rolando and Marie-Jean-Pierre Flourens' experiments on the brains of birds (chickens, cocks, ducks, hawks and pigeons), strengthened the idea of sleep as a passive process (i.e. the subtraction of wakefulness). Johannes Evangelistica Purkinje (1787–1869) – a Czechoslovakian physiologist who emphasized the importance of lower brain centres for some activities in the upper parts of the brain – was likewise inclined to believe that 'only waking – and not sleep – was an active state of the brain, with its own function' (Hobson 1995: 5–6). With 'one or two exceptions', indeed, most thinkers, up until the mid-twentieth century, regarded sleep as either an inevitable result of reduced sensory input (with the consequent diminution of brain activity and the occurrence of sleep) or the product of blood leaving (anaemia) or putting pressure (congestion) on the brain (Dement 2000: 2). No real distinction, moreover, was 'drawn between sleep and other states of quiescence such as coma, stupor, intoxication, hypnosis, anaesthesia and hibernation' (2000: 2).

The intriguing 'hypnotoxin' theory was also formulated around the turn of the twentieth century, particularly through the work of the French physiologists Rene Legendre (1912) and Henri Pieron (1913) who conducted experiments showing how blood serum extracted from sleep-deprived dogs could induce sleep in non-sleep deprived dogs. These experiments, however, were preceded by the 'toxic' claims of others such as Raymond Emil Dubois (1894) who proposed that sleep was due to carbon dioxide toxicity, and Abel Bouchard who proposed in 1886 that sleep was due to 'urotoxins' excreted in the urine during sleep (Thorpy 1991).

Mention should also be made, at this point, of various 'inhibitory' (reflex) theories of sleep, particularly those expounded by the likes of Charles Édouard Brown-Sequard in 1889, and, perhaps most notably, Ivan Petrovich Pavlov (1849–1936) in the early twentieth century. Pavlov's famous experiments with dogs, in this respect, did not simply end when the bell rang and the dog duly salivated. He also showed how a continuous stimulus induced drowsiness or sleep in his canine subjects. It is clear, Pavlov stated, on the basis of this and subsequent research (Pavlov 1923, 1927, 1928), that 'our daytime work represents the sum total of excitations which entail a certain amount of exhaustion, and the latter, carried to a certain point, calls forth automatically. . .the condition of inhibition, accompanied by sleep' (Pavlov quoted in Kleitman 1963/1939: 346). Sleep, in other words, was a process of 'spreading cortical inhibition': a kind of domino effect of fatigued brain cells turning off one by one until sleep ensued. Vladimir Michailovitch Bechterev (1932) likewise believed that sleep was a 'reflex' that may be evoked (Thorpy 1991: xxvi), which itself resembled the views of Édouard Claparede, who proclaimed in 1905 that sleep was an 'instinct' (Hobson 1995: 107).

Another key figure who clearly stands out in the history of sleep research, is Constantin von Economo (1876–1931), a Viennese neurologist who himself was influenced by the work of Pieron and Pavlov[1]. The brainstem, von Economo reasoned, based on his own clinical observations and experimental work, does not simply support or regulate wakefulness, it also supports or regulates sleep (von Economo 1930). The waking-centre and the sleep-centre, he speculated, echoing Pieron's theories, worked via chemical substances (Hobson 1995; Kleitman 1963/1939).

The major 'breakthrough' in the early twentieth century, however, came from the German psychiatrist Johannes (Hans) Berger (1873–1941). His recording of electrical activity of the human brain, beginning in 1928, clearly demonstrated distinctive and recognisable wave forms according to activities and events such as closing of the eyes, concentrating, and loud noises – observations preceded by the important work of Camillo Golgi (1843–1926) and Santiago Ramon y Cajal (1852–1934) on the nervous system and the demonstration of electrical rhythms in the brains of animals by the Scottish physiologist Richard Caton in 1875 (Thorpy 1991). Berger (1930) correctly inferred that the signals he received, which he called 'Elekrenkephalogramms' (the English translation, of course, being 'electroencephalograms'), originated in the brain, thereby setting in train what later came to be an effective if not essential tool for the scientific (read psychophysiological) recording of 'sleep'[2]. The relevance of the electroencephalogram (EEG) to the study of sleep, however, was not immediately apparent. It was not until 1935 that the utility of the EEG as a sleep recording device was successfully demonstrated through the work of Alfred Loomis and colleagues in New York (Loomis et al. 1935a,b, cited in Morgan 1987: 5). This, in conjunction with subsequent research at Harvard University and the University of Chicago between 1937–39 (see, for example, Blake et al 1939), helped establish all the major elements of brain wave patterns in sleep (Dement 2000: 3). Sleep, as a consequence, was duly classified or divided into five distinct stages from A to E (Thorpy 1991: xxviii).

The path ahead, however, was far from simple or straightforward. The 'passive' theory of sleep, indeed, received a further boost in the mid-1930s through the work of the Belgian physiologist Frederick Bremer. Bremer (1935) concluded on the basis of his studies of brain wave patterns in two cat 'cerveauisole preparations' (i.e. transactions of the mid brain), that a functional 'deafferentation' of the cerebral cortex occurred in sleep, which in everyday parlance meant that he favoured the concept of sleep as a reduction of activity or a suppression of the incessant flux of nerve impulses essential for the maintenance of the waking state. Sleep, in short, was 'idling, slow synchronized "resting" neuronal activity' (Dement 2000: 3).

Further support for Bremer's theory came through other 'stimulation' experiments, such as Walter Rudolph Hess and colleagues' (1952) stimulation of the thalamus of waking cats with low-frequency pulses which induced sleep (Hobson 1995: 17). Guiseppe Moruzzi and Horace W. Magoun also published an influential paper in 1949. Their theory, based on experiments involving high-frequency electrical stimulation through electrodes implanted in the brainstem, concerned the '*ascending* reticular activating system', which to all intents and purposes, Dement (2000: 3) comments, amounted to an *active* theory of wakefulness and a *passive* theory of sleep.

Other more important developments, nonetheless, were only a few years away: developments, in the early 1950s, that quite literally set sleep science on a new track.

The 'discovery' of REM: the dawn of modern-day sleep science?

Although observations had previously been made on rapid eye movement during sleep – notably in the later part of the nineteenth century (see Thorpy 1991) – the 'discovery' or identification of the discrete organismic state known as rapid eye movement (REM) occurred in the early 1950s; a critical discovery, the significance of which was little noted in the wider community of sleep researchers at the time. Nathaniel Kleitman, the so-called 'father' of modern day sleep science, had already published a land-mark monograph entitled *Sleep and Wakefulness* in 1939 and his early work on sleep deprivation (Kleitman 1927), as a physiologist at the University of Chicago, had already cast doubt on the hypnotoxin theory, noting how levels of sleepiness varied during the day; a finding that was incompatible with a cumulative build-up of sleep-inducing hynotoxins in the blood or brain (Dement 2000). Kleitman also believed at this time, in keeping with deafferentation theory, that sleep was brought about by a reduction of peripheral stimulation due to fatigue. 'There is not a single fact about sleep', Kleitman proclaimed in the first (1939) edition of his *opus magnum*, 'that cannot be equally well interpreted as a let down of wakefulness'.

In 1951, Kleitman asked Eugene Aserinsky, a graduate student in physiology at the University of Chicago, to observe the eye movement of sleeping infants, including that of his own son. After describing the apparent rhythm in eye motility, Kleitman and Aserinsky decided to look for a similar pattern of occurrences in adults. In doing so, they developed the method of electro-oculography (EOG), which revealed a major difference between the rapid burst of motility and the slow eye movement at sleep onset. After further studies based on awakenings when rapid eye movements were present or not present, in order to elicit dream recall, Aserinsky and Kleitman concluded that REM was associated with dreaming: a finding which Dement (2000: 6) describes as nothing short of a 'breakthrough', if not the beginnings of sleep research as we know it today[3].

The seminal Aserinsky and Kleitman paper was published in *Science* in 1953, the year of Watson and Crick's discovery of DNA, but attracted little attention at the time within the scientific community. In fact, no publications on the subject, Dement (2000) reports, appeared from any other laboratory until 1959. These insights, nevertheless, were carried forward by Dement and Kleitman through continuous all-night sleep recordings throughout typical nights of sleep. A total of 126 nights from 33 subjects were observed by means of a simplified pattern of EEG recordings, thereby building up a systematic body of data on the intricate pattern or architecture of a typical night's sleep (Dement and Kleitman 1957). Although this sequence of regular variations has been observed thousands of times in hundreds of sleep laboratories all over the world, the original description, Dement (2000: 7) proudly proclaims, has remained essentially unchanged:

> The usual sequence was that after the onset of sleep, the EEG progressed fairly rapidly to Stage 4, which persisted for varying amounts of time, generally about 30 minutes, and then a lightening took place. While the progression from wakefulness to Stage 4 at the beginning of the cycle was almost invariably through a continuum of change, the lightening was usually abrupt and coincident with a body movement or series of movements. After the termination of Stage 4, there was generally a short period of Stage 2 or 3 which gave way to Stage 1 and Rapid Eye Movements. When the first eye movement period ended, the EEG again progressed through a continuum of change to Stage 3 or 4 which persisted for a time and then lightened, often abruptly, with body movement to Stage 2 which again gave way to Stage 1 and the second Rapid Eye Movement period.
>
> (Dement and Kleitman 1957: 679)

This cyclical variation occurred repeatedly throughout the night at intervals of approximately 90–100 minutes from the end of one period of REM to the next. In contrast to the prevailing notion of sleep as a single state, moreover, Dement and Kleitman characterised:

> . . . the EEG during REM periods as 'emergent stage 1' as opposed to 'descending stage 1' at the onset of sleep. The percentage of the total time occupied by REM sleep was between 20 and 25% and the periods of REM sleep tended to be shorter in the early cycles of the night. Variations in this picture of all-night sleep have been seen over and over in normal human beings of both genders, in widely varying environments and cultures, and, to all intents and purposes, across the lifespan.
>
> (Dement 2000: 7).

Sleep, then, from this time onwards, 'could no longer be thought of as a time of brain inactivity and EEG slowing'. A 'basic duality of sleep', in short, scientifically or organismically speaking, was now firmly established through the REM/NREM divide – with standardised terminology, techniques and scoring system for sleep stages of human subjects (cf. Rechtschaffen and Kales 1968) – and the notion of sleep as a 'passive' state (i.e. the ascending reticular system theory) duly challenged if not totally demolished (Dement 2000: 8).

Other key developments, at this time, include Michel Jouvet's (Jouvet et al 1959, Jouvet and Mounier 1960) demonstration of REM sleep-related muscle atonia (i.e. loss of muscle tone) in cats – a finding preceded by Freud's reputed observations on the paralysis of skeletal muscles during dream sleep in 1895 (Thorpy 1991: xxvii) – and his related work on the role of serotonin and serotonic neurons in the brain stem; see Jouvet (1999; 1965) for a detailed account of *The Paradox of Sleep*[4].

By the 1960s then, it was possible to define REM sleep as a 'completely separate organismic state characterised by cerebral activation, active motor inhibition, and, of course, an association with dreaming' (Dement 2000: 8). REM sleep, indeed, is deeply 'paradoxical', given the EEG suggests light sleep whilst the individual is in fact quite deeply asleep; hence the term 'paradoxical', 'active' or 'dreaming sleep' (Morgan 1987: 8). In short, the 'fundamental duality of sleep', scientifically speaking, was seen to be 'an established fact' (Dement 2000: 8).

These developments, in turn, were augmented through the work of researchers at the Max Planck Institute in Germany who, continuing the tradition of Jean Jacques d'ortous de Mairan's first 'chronobiological experiments' way back in 1729, were able to demonstrate that the rhythms of sleeping and awakening are set by an 'internal clock'. The real 'breakthroughs' on this front, however, came through research in the 1970s and 1980s which demonstrated the role of bright light in resetting the 'circadian cycle' (see, for example, Czeisler et al 1986) – the term circadian derives from the Latin *circa* (near or close to) and *dias* (day) – and the identification of the locus of this 'biological clock' deep in the brain in two 'pinhead sized clusters of nerve cells called the suprachiasmic nuclei, or SCN' (Dement with Vaughan 2000: 87–98). Again the implications of these findings have been regarded as 'far reaching' within sleep science, not least in establishing beyond doubt that being surrounded by electric light in the evening – what Coren (1996) dubs 'Edison's curse' – 'pushes our biological clocks around', if not throws a 'dangerous wrench into the human clockworks' (Dement with Vaughan 2000: 100).

The work of the Stamford group of sleep scientists, including Dement, has also resulted in what he himself unashamedly describes as a 'beautiful' model of the sleep–waking process, namely the 'opponent-process model' which explains 'why people usually can stay awake or fall asleep when they want to and why sometimes this is impossible' (Dement with Vaughan 2000: 79). According to this model, the 'biological sleep drive' that causes us to fall asleep and to remain asleep through the night is:

> . . . continuously active, even when we are awake. In fact, when we are awake, the homeostatic sleep drive is steadily increasing. Opposing this tendency is the alerting action of the biological clock. In contrast to sleep homeostasis, the process in our brain that fosters wakefulness and

sustained alertness is not active continuously. For humans and other diurnal animals, the clock-dependent alerting process is active in the daytime and inactive at night, with lowered activity in the afternoon. The push and pull of these opposing processes allows us to stay up all day and sleep all night. In summary, the main reason why we do not fall asleep as soon as we have been awake for a few hours is that the homeostatic sleep drive is strongly held at bay by the independent internal stimulation of the biological clock. The main reason that we can sleep through the night is that we have accumulated sufficient sleep debt during the day so that the unopposed homeostatic process is free to operate all night long.

(Dement with Vaughan 2000: 79–80)

These and many other developments in sleep science in the recent past have culminated in what is perhaps the boldest statement of all, by the neuropsychiatrist Allan Hobson, namely that 'more has been learned about sleep in the past 60 years, than in the preceding 6,000 years' (1995: 1). 'In this short period of time', Hobson continues, 'researchers have discovered that sleep is a dynamic behaviour, not simply the absence of waking, sleep is a special activity of the brain, controlled by elaborate and precise mechanisms' (1995: 1).

This may well be so, but important questions remain nonetheless, including the precise mechanisms of sleep and what is perhaps the trickiest matter of all, namely 'what is sleep *for*' (the function(s) of sleep, that is to say), which is the subject of much research, speculation and debate to the present day[5]. Another important question, of course – the flip side of these debates in fact – concerns what happens when we don't sleep, and how long we can do without it.

Dead tired: (record-breaking) experiments in sleep deprivation

A number of studies and experiments may be pointed to on the sleep deprivation front, both human and non-human. As far as animals go, for example, perhaps the most striking recent demonstration of sleep deprivation is to be found in the work of Allan Rechtschaffen and colleagues who reported, in 1989, that when controlled and sustained, it was 'uniformly fatal' in rats. After a week to ten days, the skin of the rats paws became ulcerated and the animal began to experience weight loss despite soaring food intake. The capacity to regulate body temperature and immune function was also lost, resulting in death within four weeks (Hobson 1995: 115; see also Kleitman's early experiments with puppies, 1927).

Obviously nothing so severe or deadly has been attempted on humans, torture or punishment notwithstanding (see Chapter 4, this book), but a number of studies of *total* sleep deprivation of varying duration have been conducted since the late nineteenth century (Hobson 1995). As for the effect, this of course depends on when and what precisely you are looking at. Humans, Hobson comments, for better or worse, seem to have a 'great capacity to endure sleep deprivation and to compensate for ensuing sleepiness'. Thus whilst:

> . . . hallucinations and illusions do occur, they are quite rare before 60 hours of deprivation. Reflexes are generally unimpaired, although tremors, eye position instability and reduced pain thresholds all denote functional neurological changes. Heart rate, blood pressure, respiration and temperature measures show only minimal changes after up to 160 hours of deprivation.
>
> (1995: 111)

This, however, is clearly no recommendation as far as sleep deprivation is concerned. There do, nonetheless, seem to have been a few high profile cases or record breaking attempts at sleep deprivation for kicks, fun or charity; the New York DJ Peter Tripp is probably the most famous of these. Tripp, in fact, has two claims to fame, first, his invention of the top 40, second, his clocking up of a total of 201 hours of continuous wakefulness as a charity fund-raising event.

The effects, to say the least, were disturbing. After three days, Tripp became abusive and unpleasant, and by the fifth day he had started to experience audio and visual hallucinations. His dreams occluded his waking thoughts and he began to see spiders crawling from his shoes. He also became increasingly paranoid, convinced that people were drugging his food, and was very nearly run over at one point after running out into the road. The changes, in turn, were accompanied by a decline in body temperature, and his brain pattern on the last evening resembled that of sleeping person even though he was 'awake'. Finally, after 201 hours, he fell into a deep sleep of approximately 24 hours. When he awoke, however, his personality, according to friends and family, was said to have changed for the worse, due perhaps to the amphetamines he had taken to get him through the long ordeal. He subsequently left his wife, lost his job and became a drifter (Dement with Vaughan 2000).

Tripp, to be sure, did not break the world record, but a San Diego high-school student by the name of Randy Gardner did, clocking up an incredible 264 hours of continuous wakefulness, thereby beating the previous Guinness Book of Records total of 260 hours. At first he found staying awake easy. By the third day however it became increasingly difficult, especially at night. Shaking and urging him on was the only way to avoid him falling asleep. Finally, after 264 hours of wakefulness or sleep deprivation, Gardner slept for a total of 14 hours and 40 minutes, with no apparent ill effects, either physical or mental, short or long term (Dement with Vaughan 2000). Unlike Tripp, it seems, Gardner emerged relatively unscathed, with only the press to answer to and the cheers of his schoolmates.

Researchers have subsequently studied the effects of *limited* sleep rather than total sleep deprivation. They have also, following the division of sleep, sought to investigate whether deprivation of a specific sort has specific consequences: findings, amongst other things, which clearly suggest that 'the brain "knows" it needs to make up for lost REM and that it also knows how much it needs to make up' (Hobson 1995: 111–13).

We shall return to these issues in Chapters 4 and 5 in the context of broader debates as to whether or not society is (chronically) sleep deprived, and links between sleep, health and risk. For the moment, however, it is to that other prime cause of sleep disturbance, disruption or deprivation that we now turn, namely the 'problems', 'pains', 'perils', if not 'pathologies' of sleep. How did our ancestors fare on this count? What sense did they make of these trials and tribulations of sleep? And what remedies did they turn to?

The 'trials' and 'tribulations' of sleep: prophecies, premonitions and precursors of modern-day 'sleep medicine'

People have doubtless always had sleep 'problems', in one form or another. Observations, explanations and treatments for the 'pains' if not the 'pathologies' of sleep, in this respect, stretch way back to the dim and distant past, as do associations between sleep, health and hygiene (see for example Dannenfeldt 1986 and Chapters 2 and 5 in this book). A rudimentary understanding of 'insomnia' – a term derived from the Latin words *in* (meaning not) and *somnus* (meaning sleep) – and sleepiness, for example, was certainly evident in ancient times. Treatments or remedies for sleep problems have likewise been practised throughout the ages: from praying, divination, dream interpretation and appeasement of the gods, through blood letting, diet, exercise, music and meditation, to medications such as theria (derived from plants and animals, including snake flesh), opium (laudanum) and mid-nineteenth-century hypnotics such as bromide (Thorpy 1991). Acupuncture and moxibustion, together with herbal medicines, massage and breathing exercises, also date back to ancient Chinese times and continue to the present day as alternatives, complements or companions to Western biomedical prescriptions for sleep 'problems' (Thorpy 1991; see also Chapter 5 in this book).

Clearly one needs to distinguish here, at an early stage, between sleep disorders or pathologies as such, and 'problems' consequent upon other physical or mental afflictions, such as pain of various sorts: a distinction more pertinent to present times perhaps, particularly over the past 50 years or so where differentiation between the causes and complications of sleepiness has flourished, but important to bear in mind nonetheless in sifting and sorting the past from the present.

As far as the past descriptions of sleep problems or disorders are concerned, a variety of sources and insights are evident that presage or predate current clinical or pathological concerns. The clinical features of sleep apnoea, for example, Kryger (1983) claims, were clearly evident if not explicitly formulated in antiquity[6]. Dionysius the Heracleote, son of Clearchus the tyrant (born in approximately 360BC in the era of Alexander the Great), is a case in point. By all accounts, Dionysius was a gluttonous, obese man who lived the life of luxury and over-indulgence. As a consequence, he was afflicted with shortened breath (dyspnoea) and bouts or fits of choking. When he slept, it was impossible to wake him without piercing his flesh with pins (which first had to penetrate many layers of fat to produce the desired result): a treatment designed, in part, to keep Dionysius breathing. Dionysius, indeed, reputedly lived in fear of suffocation from fat. Several features of this case, Kryger comments, suggest that Dionysius had sleep apnoea, notably 'obesity, problems with breathing ("a fat hog lying upon the snout"), sleepiness and the fact he was difficult to arouse' (1983: 2301). The disease, moreover, he contends, was 'not so rare in antiquity' (1983: 2301; see also Lavie 1986 on historical accounts of sleep apnoea, Netzer 2002 on 'snoring in the ancient world', de Montaigne 1991/1572 on the snoring of Emperor Otho and the great Cato, and Wadd's 1822/1816 'Cursory Remarks on Corpulence: or obesity considered as a disease').

Other important reference points here, of course, include the likes of Shakespeare, whose works provide an extraordinarily rich source of insight into the trials and tribulations of sleep. Many of Shakespeare's characters were troubled by afflictions that latter-day sleep scientists and clinicians would dub or describe as sleep apnoea, somnambulism, somniloquoy, insomnia and nightmares. Sleep, to be sure, was a 'blessing' for Shakespeare – 'Sleep that knots up the ravell'd sleave of care. . .sore labour's bath . . .. Balm of hurt minds . . . chief nourisher in life's feast' – but one, it seems, that all too often evaded the players of his parts. We see this, for example, quite clearly in the somnambulism and somniloquoy of Lady Macbeth, the sleep apnoea of Falstaff in Henry IV, the insomnia of Henry IV and Macbeth, and the nightmares of Richard III (Furman et al 1997). In Hamlet, moreover, in an echo of ancient Greek mythology, sleep is linked to death, and dreams themselves are taken to symbolize experiences after death (Furman et al 1997: 1172): 'To die – to sleep – To sleep! Perchance to dream. Ay there's the rub; For in that sleep of death what dreams may come, When we have shuffled off this mortal coil, Must give us pause. There's the respect, That makes calamity of so long life. . .' (Act III Scene i; see also Chapter 3, this book).

Coleridge is another great literary reference point here as far as the 'pains of sleep go', including a poem bearing this very title. Throughout his lifetime, Coleridge suffered from many types of illness, often opium-related through his use or withdrawal from the drug. Sleep, as Ford notes, became a 'physical catalogue of discomfort and terror' for Coleridge, who felt him-self '"afflicted" in every possible way', leaving him terrified at the very thought of going to bed (Ford 2004: 112). Consider, for example, Coleridge's (1971/1820–25) letter to Thomas Allsop on 1st July 1820, in which he confesses that it is the 'howling Wilderness of sleep that I dread'. Another letter, dated 4th July 1820, to his son Derwent, is equally telling of these afflictions:

> . . .during the day or as a long as I am up, I am calm or at all events can manage what I feel – But – I cannot tell why – as soon as my head is on the pillow, my thoughts become their own masters, in spite of every effort to go to sleep with indifferent trains of thinking & tho' I do not go to bed till I am down-right weary of holding myself up & continue reading & trying to interest my intellect or fancy in the subject to the last moment. Last night, however, I screamed out but once only in my sleep, & my stomach felt but in a very slight degree sore after I awoke – the exceeding order & wild Swedenborghean rationality of the Image of my Dreams, whenever I have been in any great affliction, so that they haunt me for days – & the odd circumstance that these dreams are always accompanied by profuse weeping in my sleep toward morning, & probably not very long before I wake – for my pillow is often quite wet: (for the screaming fits take place in the first sleep, & from dreams that are either frightful or mere imageless sensation of affright & leave no traces). . .

The letter was duly signed 'Your afflicted & loving Father, S.T Coleridge'.

Coleridge, as this extract attests, drew 'strong connections between his dream life and his (diseased) bodily life', particularly the gastric system and the nervous ganglionic seen as 'attaining "paramouncy" over the brain (the "cerebral") while he was sleeping' (Ford 2004: 112). There were, in other words, complex associations between psyche and soma during sleep, for Coleridge, who coined the term 'psychosomatic' to describe them. He also, however, believed that dreams could be caused by spirits (Ford 2004: 118–19).

Perhaps the most widely recognised and celebrated literary insights into sleep disorders, nonetheless, can be found in the works of one Charles Dickens. As with Shakespeare, Dickens' work covers a wide range of what would subsequently come to be known and clinically described as sleep disorders; an interest prompted by his own periodic bouts of insomnia (Cosnet 1997). The most famous of these descriptions, no doubt, published in *The Posthumous Papers of the Pickwick Club* (Dickens 1909/1836–7), concerns the fat boy Joe, a character apparently based on a bully boy called

James Budden from Dickens' own past. Joe has a voracious appetite, is obese and suffers from somnolence or excessive sleepiness. He also snores loudly. Most of the time, indeed, Joe is either eating or sleeping. So legendary is this Dickensian description in fact, that sleep apnoea itself, in a paper published in the *American Journal of Medicine* in 1956 (Burwell et al 1956), was dubbed the 'Pickwickian syndrome'; an association which has stuck ever since. Elsewhere, Dickens alludes to the 'choke and snore' of a coffee stall holder in *The Uncommercial Traveller* (1973/1860) and the 'slight difficulty in respiration, such as a carpenter encounters when he is planing and comes to a knot' – a description of John Willet's breathing when asleep in *Barnaby Lodge* (Cosnet 1997: 201).

Dickens' observations on sleep problems or disorders, however, do not end here. Many of Dickens' characters, like he himself, suffered from (occasional) bouts of insomnia. He also described, in books such as *David Copperfield, Our Mutual Friend, Oliver Twist, Domby and Son*, and *A Christmas Carol*, various hypnagogic states, cases of restless leg syndrome, perils of sleep paralysis, as well as the horrors of nightmares and episodes of sleep-walking. Most of these observations, Cosnet (1997) remarks, have subsequently proved to be remarkably accurate in the light of current knowledge, and must have been based on Dickens' own experience. He also, like many other prominent, creative people, found 'advantage' in his insomnia: itself providing ample opportunity for night walks in London, and affording further time for 'reflection and invention of plots, characters and dialogue for his novels' (Cosnet 1997: 204).

Literature, of course, did not completely steal the march on medicine, as far as the description or documentation of sleep disorders were concerned. The neurologist Thomas Willis, for example, in his aforementioned book *The London Practice of Physick* (1692), documented many problems and disorders of sleep, or the 'irregularities and morbid exorbitancies of sleep and watching' as he termed it, including restless leg syndrome, nightmares (or the 'incubus') and insomnia (or the 'watching evil'), alongside 'instructions concerning opiates, or medicines that cause sleep, with their good and ill effects; together with prescripts of them'. As regards instructions and prescripts for curing the 'watching evil' and the 'watching coma', for example, Willis clearly acknowledges the need to distinguish this as a symptom of some other disease (e.g. fever, frenzy, mania, colic or gout) and continual waking or the watching evil as a 'disease of itself' in which people, the 'destitute of sleep', are 'forced to have recourse to opiates, which sometimes they use daily, and in large dose without hurt' (1692: 402–3). The latter, he claimed, in keeping with his previously outlined explanation of sleep, was due to 'Spirits not thereby torpid, or wearied, or exhausted', spirits sufficiently refreshed and 'freed from the fetters or Nervous Liquour: Vigorous exert themselves and are expanded everyway, and especially from the middle part of the Brain to its circumference' (1692: 403).

Further 'advances' were also made in the clinical description of sleep disorders in the nineteenth century. William Wadd, for example, Surgeon Extraordinary to the King, wrote an instructive monograph in 1816, entitled *Cursory Remarks on Corpulence*, noting *inter alia* how breathing may be impaired by obesity and how obese people become sleepy (Kryger 1983). William Alexander Hammond, the noted American Physician, also produced a book, entitled *Sleep and its Derangements* in 1869, based on a series of publications concerning insomnia; whilst Silas Weir Mitchell (1829–1914) wrote a number of clinical articles on sleep, including abnormal breathing during sleep, nocturnal epilepsy, night terrors and the effects of stimulants on insomnia (Thorpy 1991: xxv; see, for example, Weir Mitchell 1890; see also Dana 1884). Another interesting historical source is to be found buried in the pages of the *Birmingham Medical Review* in 1882. The article, written by one W.E. Green M.R.C.S., bears the title 'Sleeplessness, its causes and treatment'[7]. It opens as follows:

> For some years now I have been much interested in the subject of sleeplessness, convinced as I am that it is one of the most troublesome symptoms which either a medical man has to encounter, or a patient has to endure. The condition in the patient often amounts to one of actual misery; while the medical man is troubled on account of the difficulty he frequently experiences in successfully combating the affection.
>
> (1882: 161).

From the experiments of various observers, Green proclaims, it 'now seems placed beyond reasonable doubt that sleep is a condition of physiological cerebral anaemia' (1882: 162). As to the varieties of sleeplessness or insomnia, a number are considered and discussed: from insomnia produced by *cold (feet)*, through *dyspeptic insomnia, cerebral excitement* and *pyrexial sleeplessness*, to *anaemic insomnia* or anaemic sleeplessness, *gouty insomnia* and *nervous insomnia*. Some of the 'commoner hypnotics in use' are then listed, including: *alcohol* (said to be of 'great value' in producing sleep, particularly in old people, and those who suffer from cold extremities after going to bed), *bromide of potassium, cannabis indica, chloral, croton chloral, hyoscyamus* and *lupuline, ether* and *chloroform, opium* (adjudged to be 'one of the most useful hypnotics we have'), together with *warm* or *cold bathing*, and *bodily exercise*. There are also, we are told, some *'mental means'* of attaining repose, including 'abstracting the mind from the various cares of this life by music'. Such 'diversions of the mind', Green concludes:

> . . .cannot be too highly recommended from a physiological point of view, and whether persons or families make their selection upon higher or lower grounds, this is not the place to discuss their choice.
>
> (1882: 174)

As for the sleep of doctors themselves, Alexander Hunter famously proclaimed in his 1808 edition of *Men and Manners*, the 'conscientious physician' was more than likely to suffer disturbed sleep as a result of anxiety for his patients[8].

Perhaps the greatest clinical contribution, however, as far as nineteenth-century studies of sleep disorders are concerned, pertains to the first clinical description of 'narcolepsy' as an independent disease entity in 1880 by Jean Baptiste Eduard Gelineau (1828–1906), a French physician, who derived the term from the Greek words *narcosis* (meaning benumbing) and *lepsis* (meaning to overtake). Initially, in his classic paper of 1880, published in the *Gazette des Hospitaux*, Gelineau provides a detailed description of a 38-year-old male wine barrel retailer who had sleep attacks and associated falls – the latter of which was termed 'astasia' but subsequently renamed cataplexy by Richard Hennenberg in 1916. Gelineau also went on, the following year, to describe fourteen further cases of narcolepsy, distinguishing between an idiopathic form and one related to other illnesses (Culebras 1999; Passouant 1981; Thorpy and Yager 1991: 83). Again, however, as with other sleep disorders, Gelineau's clear and detailed clinical description of narcolepsy was not altogether new. Several patients, Thorpy (1991: xxv) comments, had been previously described in the 1860s and 1870s.

These clinical insights, together with other seminal twentieth-century works such as Pieron's *Le Probleme Physiologique Du Sommeil* in 1913, Kleitman's aforementioned *Sleep and Wakefulness* in 1939 (1963/1939), and the further elaboration of existing or 'newly discovered' conditions such as 'central' sleep apnoea (i.e. the inability to breath) in 1962 – also known as 'Ondine's curse' after the water nymph in Jean Giraudoux's play *Ondine* – helped set the stage for the latter-day development of 'sleep medicine' in the closing decades of the twentieth century.

Likewise, sleep medications were undergoing significant *changes* during this time period. The first reported medication specifically used as a hypnotic, for example, was bromide, introduced in the mid-nineteenth century, followed by other sedative-hypnotics such as chloral hydrate, paraldehyde, urethane and sulfanol. In 1903, however, the barbiturate barbital was introduced. Barbiturates, including amobarbital, penobarbital, secobarbital and phenobarbital, subsequently became the treatment of choice and were used quite commonly until the 1960s, when safety concerns and new therapeutics, notably the introduction of benzodiazepine hypnotics, resulted in a decline in prescriptions. Benzodiazepines subsequently replaced barbiturates in the late 1970s. Increased physician and public concern about the disadvantages of chronic hypnotic usage in the 1980s, however, resulted in a decline in the use of these drugs; developments in part associated with a recognition that insomnia was a *symptom* rather than a diagnosis, with treatment duly redirected to the underlying physical or psychological causes

(Thorpy 1991: xxx). The introduction of a new class of supposedly safer medications in the 1990s provides yet another means at (sleep) medicine's disposal for the treatment of insomnia, with new medications currently in development.

The latter day development of sleep clinics if not 'sleep medicine' is something we shall return to and explore more fully in Chapter 5. The key point for present purposes is that important historical precursors can be found here concerning the problems or pains, if not the pathologies, of sleep, both literary and scientific in kind, including the likes of Shakespeare, Coleridge and Dickens. The systematic clinical description or 'discovery' of sleep disorders, in this respect, may well be a recent phenomenon, but this in no way should blind us to what has gone before: a history, it seems, written in many registers, some more medical or scientific than others.

But what about dreams and dreaming?

To sleep perchance to dream: the royal road to the unconscious?

This, as we know, is first and foremost a book about sleep rather than about dreams or dreaming. It would, however, be remiss or just plain wrong to neglect dreams altogether, save for the fleeting references glimpsed here and there in the foregoing pages. The history of dreams and dreaming is a rich and fascinating one. Dreams may well depend on sleep, but it is dreams, for understandable reasons perhaps, which have historically received most attention, relatively speaking: their meaning and significance the source of endless wonder, worry and wisdom.

Again there are many historical points of reference here as far as the interpretation, explanation and uses of dreams are concerned, from Ancient Egyptian, Assyrian-Babylonian dream prophecies and Judaeo-Christian Biblical references, to Galen's Treatise *Diagnosis from Dreams*; the Greek centres of dream 'incubation', particularly the oracle of Asclepius at Epidaurus, where medical 'cures' were effected from the fifth century BC onwards, to Artemidorous of Daldis *Oneirocritica* (the fortune-teller's guide to dream interpretation from the second century AD onwards); Aristotle's treatise 'on dreams' to Descartes' (1996/1641) doubts about the (shaky) distinction between dreams and our waking state, and Hobbes' (1985/1651) dismissal of the divine, diabolic or even humoral origin of dreams, to Romanticism's love affair with dreams as a source of creative insight and inspiration, including von Schubert's *Symbolism of Dreams* (1968/1814), and the Marquis Leon Hervey de Saint Deny's (1982/1867) *Dreams and How to Guide Them*. All this, moreover, without any mention of Freud or modern-day debates on the very nature and meaning(lessness) of dreams, both scientific and non-scientific in kind.

As this suggests, attitudes to dreams across the centuries:

> . . .were part of a whole package of conceptions of the body, the soul, the moral and the nature of God: and they underwent a major transformation with the new understandings of the world developed by thinkers such as Hobbes and Descartes. If dream theory had remained fairly constant from the ancients to the Renaissance, with Artemidorous's *Oneirocritica*, printed in Latin in 1518 and disseminated in vernacular language across Europe, still the authoritative manual of interpretation, dreams were nonetheless part of a simmering cauldron of debate about the divine and the diabolic, illusion and reality, which were eventually to contribute to a great deal to the intellectual shifts for the Enlightenment.
>
> (Pick and Roper 2004: 5)

These transformations, however, were far from linear or straightforward. Repeatedly, indeed, within the history of the developing 'interiorisation' of dreams, we see 'more complex oscillations and movements, shifting "viewpoints" within periods and sometimes within the same oeuvre' (Pick and Roper 2004: 7): a case, in other words, of 'unsettling movements back and forth; at one moment the dream may be construed as a phenomenon intruding from outside. . .at other points, even in contemporary works or passages of the same text, the dream may be conceived quite differently. . .each "presence" to be integrated with – seen as a product of – the psychic life of the subject' (2004: 7).

I will not dwell on these manifold meanings and references to dreams across the ages. Nor will I immerse myself in the deeper philosophical quagmire of debate, fascinating as it is, as to whether or not a firm distinction can be drawn between dreaming and waking (the Cartesian problem), whether dreams are experiences we have whilst sleeping or mere fabrications we make up on waking – a seemingly crazy thesis posed by philosophers such as Malcolm (1959) and Dennett (1978) – or the equally tricky question, stretching at least as far back as Augustine, as to whether dreams can be 'sinful' or 'immoral' (see Flanagan 2000, for example, for an excellent account of these issues).

Let me, instead, whilst duly acknowledging this broader canvas of dreams and dreaming, focus on the more familiar debate as far as the twentieth century goes, namely the Freudian interpretation of dreams and latter-day scientific challenges or assaults on this psychoanalytic edifice cum castle of dreams.

Published at the turn of the twentieth century, Freud's *Interpretations of Dreams* (1976/1900), as the foregoing discussion suggests, was both part of a long tradition of dream decipherment or interpretation, and a radical break from it. Freud's theory, as is well known, was in essence quite simple yet profound: dreams are designed to release unconscious, repressed, socially unacceptable desires and wishes, albeit in disguised form, hence the distinction between *latent* and *manifest* content. This disguised form of disclosure is crucial, not simply as the point of entry for the psychoanalyst, but as the very process that guarantees sleep: 'Dreams are the GUARDIANS of sleep and not its disturbers', Freud declares (1976/1900: 330). The censorship evident in dreams, in other words, safeguards sleep. Dreams, in turn, may be the 'royal road to the unconscious' but only with the psychoanalyst's lantern shining on their latent content *qua* 'dream-thoughts'. 'Every attempt that has hitherto been made to solve the problem of dreams', Freud states, 'has hitherto dealt directly with their *manifest* content as it is presented in our memory'. 'We [the psychoanalytic fraternity that is] are alone', he continues:

> ... in taking something else into account. We have introduced a new class of psychical material between the manifest content of dreams and the conclusions of our enquiry: namely, their *latent* content, or (as we say) the 'dream-thoughts', arrived at by our procedure. It is from these dream-thoughts and not from a dream's manifest content that we disentangle its meaning. We are thus presented with a *new task which had no previous existence*: the task, that is, of investigating relations between the manifest contents of dreams and the latent dream-thoughts, and of tracing out the process by which the latter have been changed into the former.
>
> (1976/1900: 381)

This, Flanagan comments, is compatible with the plausible evolutionary idea, which provides dreams with a 'natural biological function – the wish-release-function'. It also suggests that dreams can be a 'valuable source of self-knowledge when such knowledge is needed to alleviate neurosis' (2000: 43–4).

Freud, to be sure, placed a premium on the sexual or aggressive undertones of dreams. Dissension, nonetheless, was not far off. Jung, for example, stressed the deeper spiritual and archetypal significance of dreams (Shamadsani 2003), whilst Adler (1912) emphasized the link between dreams and self-esteem. The unconscious, moreover, was far from a total Freudian invention. Before Freud had begun his research into hysteria and dreams, for instance, British investigation based around the Society for Psychical Research – led by the likes of Henry Sidgwick, Edmund Gurney and Fredrick Myers – had already pioneered the idea of the subliminal or subconscious mind: part and parcel, as Hayward puts it, of a 'policing of dreams' in the nineteenth century, which collapsed the discordant and anomalous knowledge of dreams into the 'sanctioned narratives of the individual life history' (2004: 165, 170).

Freud's ideas, nonetheless, have been hugely influential, indelibly etching themselves on the twentieth-century if not the twenty-first-century Western psyche. This, of course, includes endorsement, revision and outright rejection.

As far as twentieth–twenty-first-century dream research goes, Hobson and colleagues provide what is perhaps the most sustained engagement and critique of Freud's theory of dreams. Freud, Hobson (2002) claims, quoting a favoured source, 'was 50 per cent right and 100 per cent wrong'. In seeking to 'unpack' this paradox, he proceeds to show that 'only experimental brain science can hope to correct any picture of ourselves based on intuition alone' (2002: 148).

As for what Freud got right, his discussion of dreams, Hobson maintains, correctly emphasised their primitive character. Dreams, that is to say, 'are indeed instigated by the release in sleep of primitive drive mechanisms of the brain'. But, Hobson hastens to add, there is 'a lot less sex than Freud assumed and a lot more of the negative emotions than he was prepared to deal with, because he placed so much emphasis on dreaming or wish fulfilment' (2002: 149).

As for what Freud got wrong, he is alleged to have adopted a 'fatally flawed assumption of disguise and censorship as the basis of dream bizzareness'. If the dream-inducing instincts are not disguised and not censored, in other words, but enter into the dream plots directly, then the 'manifest dream is the dream, is the dream, is the dream!' (Hobson 2002: 151). Hence Freud's classic distinction between manifest and latent dream content, upon which psychoanalysis depends, disappears in favour of a far simpler, less convoluted approach. We do not, in short, from this new neurophysiological science of dreaming:

> ...dream because our unconscious wishes or drives would, if undisguised, wake us up. We dream because our brains are activated during sleep, and we do so even if our primitive drives are turned on by that activation. In fact, *such drives are not concealed*. It is the *specific neurophysiological details of that activation process, not psychological defence mechanisms*, that determine the instinctive nature of dream consciousness.
>
> (Hobson 2002: 158)

Dreams then, from this perspective, wrested from the psychoanalyst's couch, are expressions of 'brain activation' and henceforth the province of brain research and sleep science. The logic here runs as follows: the study of dreaming becomes 'inextricably linked' to sleep science, which in turn is 'inextricably linked' to neurobiology, including the brain chemistry that differentiates waking and dream consciousness. This, Hobson proudly concludes, is 'a time of renaissance, a genuine revolution, and a major shift' in the scientific theory of brain and mind: 'nothing less is at stake than a scientific theory of human consciousness' (2002: 161–2).

Flanagan (2000) too, in a variant on these themes, rejects Freud's theory of manifest and latent dream content, showing how brain stem activity during sleep generates a jumbled profusion of images, memories, thoughts, emotions and desires, which the cerebral cortext then attempts to sift, sort and shape into a more or less coherent story. Whilst sleep, from this perspective, has a clear biological function and adaptive value, dreams are merely 'random side effects', 'free riders' or the 'spandrels of sleep'; 'irrelevant' from an evolutionary point of view (see also Crick and Mitchison 1983, 1995). However bizarre these narratives may be, Flanagan insists they can still shed light on our mental life, our well-being and our sense of self. Dreams, that is to say, are 'not just noise'. Some dreams, indeed, are 'self-expressive and worth attention in the project of gaining, enhancing, and refining self-knowledge. We are dreaming souls. And the brain is the seat of our soul whether we are asleep or awake' (2000: 195). Here again, then, we have a variant on the theme of Freud being partly right and wholly wrong.

Let us pass, for the moment at least, over any (counter) charge of misunderstanding or reductionism here, on Hobson's part at least, in favour of two further points about dreams and dreaming, themselves closely interrelated. The first of these, of course, embedded in these very debates, is that dreams can be pleasurable if not creative. If indeed the claims of the great and the good are to be believed, we have dreams to thank for many discoveries and works of art, from Descartes' philosophical system to Einstein's theory of relativity, Coleridge's poem 'Kubla Kahn' to Mary Shelley's *Frankenstein*, Salvador Dali's surreal landscapes to Stevenson's *Dr Jekyll and Mr Hyde*, Blake's artistic outpourings to Beatles tracks such as *Yesterday* and *Let it Be*.

This in turn leads to the second important point about different 'types' of dreams. Earlier it was suggested, following the 'discovery' of REM and the delineation of two distinct types of sleep, that dreams take place during 'emergent Stage 1' (i.e. REM sleep). It is now fairly well established, however, that dreaming occurs in the absence of REMs, including periods of 'quiet' sleep (Mavromatis 1987: 95–6; Flanagan 2000). The Dutch psychiatrist Frederick van Eeden, way before REM was discovered, proposed no less than nine different kinds of 'dream', including what he called the 'initial dream', the 'lucid dream' and the 'wrong waking up' (i.e. false or dreamt awakenings) (1913). The boundaries between these issues and various hypnagogic states (a term coined by Alfred Maury to denote pre-sleep or sleep-onset phenomena) and hypnopompic states (a term coined by Fredric Myers to denote coming or leading out of sleep phenomena) is hazy or fuzzy to say the least (see Mavromatis 1987 for a definitive account of these 'twilight', 'borderland', 'half dream' or *'prae dormitium'* phenomena and their complex relationships to other states such as out-of-body experiences [OBEs])[9].

Lucid dreaming, for example, illustrates these issues well. Usually, when we are dreaming, we are not aware we are dreaming. Lucid dreaming, in contrast, involves the conscious awareness that one is dreaming. It may also, occasionally or fleetingly, involve the ability to direct one's dreams in playful or pleasurable ways like an 'inner' theatre of the imagination. Again one may approach this weird and wonderful phenomenon from a variety of angles, both past and present. Perhaps the most notable reference, as far as the nineteenth century goes, concerns the aforementioned Marquis Leon Hervey de Saint-Deny's (anonymously published) *Dreams and How to Guide Them* (1982/1867): a work that was little known at the time. Hervey, by his own admission, had recorded thousands of his own dreams, including various hypnagogic states, and had pretty well mastered the art of lucid dreaming: an art he hoped everyone could enjoy and share in. Those that were aware of the book's existence, such as Alfred Maury and Havelock Ellis, were often sceptical, denouncing any such notion of dreaming self-consciousness. The statement 'I am asleep', as the philosopher Malcolm (1959) more recently put it, is a logical impossibility.

There are, nonetheless, scattered allusions to, if not advocates of, such lucid dream states before and after this time, including Fredrick van Eeden (who coined the term 'lucid dreams' in 1913), Frederic Myers, the occult writer Oliver Fox, and the British psychologist Mary Arnold Foster (Melechi 2003: 169–70). Even Plato, Aristotle, Augustine, Nietzsche and Freud had acknowledged the possibility of the sleeper being 'conscious of the sleeping state', so too Dickens, if not Coleridge and Shakespeare.

It was not until the late 1960s, however, that lucid dreaming became a subject of academic interest through books such as Celia Green's (1968) *Lucid Dreaming*. It gained further impetus in the late 1970s through New Age advocates and the scientific research of figures such as Keith Hearne (1990) from the University of Hull, UK, and Stephen La Berge and colleagues at Stanford University in the US: a confluence or cocktail of factors, as Melechi notes, which promise rather more than Hervey or any of his predecessors (2003: 174). See also Tart (1988) for a useful review of attempts to consciously control nocturnal dreaming.

La Berge, for example, based on a growing body of empirical evidence and collaborative studies (La Berge and Dement 1982, La Berge and Rheingold 1990; La Berge et al 1981), has demonstrated that lucid dreaming occurs during unequivocal REM sleep – the most active period of phasic rather than tonic REM – and that lucid dreaming is a 'learnable skill', if not the cheapest form of home entertainment around, with a variety of techniques available for inducing such states. This includes a procedure that La Berge terms MILD (mnemonic induction of lucid dreams), which involves things such as writing down and rehearsing dreams, saying to oneself 'the next time I am dreaming, I want to remember I am dreaming', visualizing your body lying asleep in bed, and so on (La Berge 1980, 1985). Try it yourself and see what happens. . ..

Whilst lucid dreaming, as this suggests, may be a fun pursuit or pastime, most recent scientific research has been directed toward the *use* of lucid dreaming as a treatment for nightmares, anxiety, depression and grief (Melechi 2003: 174). At the same time, transpersonal psychologists have claimed lucidity as a 'bona fide spiritual technology, a form of "deep witnessing" comparable to various forms of meditation'. Forms of lucid dreaming, moreover, have a long-standing place in Tibetan dream yoga, Hindu dream witnessing and New World Shamanism (Melechi 2003: 174). Lucid dreaming, as this suggests, has many potential uses and abuses, some more recent and some more dubious than others.

Here it seems is a fitting place to stop, as the debate about the boundaries between dreaming and waking consciousness, not to mention the possibilities of being 'sinful' or 'immoral' in one's dreams, turns full circle.

Conclusions

The purpose of this chapter has been to take a preliminary look, no more or less, at the mysteries of sleep and at attempts to unravel them, with particular reference to philosophical, scientific and literary sources, and insights into these dormant matters from ancient to modern times. Sleep, as we have seen, has been the source of much speculation and debate, including the development of chemical, vascular, neural and behavioural explanations, and a shift from 'passive' to 'active' theories with the dawn of sleep science as we know it today. What we have here, then, is a history of changing ideas, theories and explanations of sleep and dreams, including literary descriptions of the problems and pains of sleep, which take us all the way from Aristotle to Descartes, MacNish to Kleitman, Bremer to Dement, Freud to Hobson, Shakespeare to Dickens. In this respect, the social construction of sleep as an object of study and a topic of discussion and debate, within and beyond scientific circles, is clearly apparent. The landscape of sleep research, moreover, has clearly shifted in the latter part of the twentieth century from a predominant concern with the underlying mechanisms of 'normal' sleep, monitored and measured in the sleep lab, to the pathologies of sleep, treated in the sleep clinic (Kroker 2005): a topic we shall return to in Chapter 5.

So how then, sifting and sorting through all this, should we define sleep, for present purposes at least? As far as the characteristic features of sleep are concerned, two key criteria stand out above all others: first, the 'perceptual wall' sleep erects between the sleeper and the outside world (itself of course selective rather than total); second, its (rapid) reversibility compared to the irreversibility of death (Dement with Vaughan 2000). Sleep, in other words, involves a loss of consciousness to the outside world that is 'lived through'. To this we might add other important features or characteristics of sleep, such as its regular waxing and waning according to a circadian rhythm, the posture of the body (usually recumbent), the place where it occurs (usually, though not always, a bed or similar device in a bedroom or secluded spot), and the relative immobility it entails (Martin 2003; Kleitman 1963/1939). Technically or organismically speaking, as we have seen, there are two distinct types of sleep, namely REM and NREM, the former of more recent origin, in evolutionary terms, tied to the most active, lucid or vivid form of dreaming; a claim, it should be emphasised, which in no way denies the possibility of other NREM forms of dreaming.

Sleep, as this suggests, is a complex behaviour or practice that cannot solely or simply be equated or conflated with the closing of our eyes, the partaking of rest, retiring to bed, or even the dreaming of dreams. I may, for example, lie in bed all night with my eyes tightly shut, without getting a wink of sleep. It is possible furthermore to sleep with one's eyes wide open. We are also quite 'busy' when we are asleep, whether we are dreaming or not, including the continuation of vital processes such as respiration, heartbeat and digestion. Sleep, from this perspective, is far from simply restful (in)activity. Although sleep cannot be directly willed, 'descending' or 'coming over us', it does nonetheless involve important 'learnt', 'habitual' and 'reflexive' components, which themselves are socially, culturally and historically variable: a point we shall return to and elaborate more fully in subsequent chapters.

Whether or not sleep is a welcome or unwelcome 'release' from the conscious demands of the waking world, of course, depends on your perspective. Whichever way one looks at it, relations between sleep and wakefulness are complex, with a variety of intermediate states 'in between'. The statement 'I am asleep', in this respect, is not quite so philosophically absurd or logically impossible as it may seem, particularly when lucid dreaming, amongst other things, is taken into account.

As to whether or not sleep is a distinctly human trait, the answer of course is 'No'. We are, it seems, in very good company when it comes to sleep, although the precise nature of sleep, in this respect, is variable or species specific. Adopting a broad definition of 'sleep', one can safely say that all mammals, birds, amphibians, reptiles, fish and insects, so far studied, have been found to partake, in one way or another. The two-toed sloth, for example, devotes approximately twenty hours per day, or more than eighty per cent of its life to sleep. Cows, goats, donkeys, horses, sheep, deer and giraffes, on the other hand, get by on a minimum of three to four hours per day, elephants on about six hours, thereby placing us humans somewhere in the middle of the spectrum (Martin 2003: 12). Some creatures, given their habitat, have invented ingenious ways to sleep. The dolphin, for instance, cunningly sleeps on one side of its brain at a time, thereby enabling it to continually resurface for air whilst 'asleep'.

For all this, the precise function of sleep, from an evolutionary perspective, is still pretty much a mystery, particularly when the vulnerability of sleeping creatures is taken into account. There are good reasons for thinking that sleep has adaptive value and serves a proper biological function, including restorative/conservatory/building and information processing roles (Flanagan 2000; Hobson 1995). Prolonged sleep deprivation, as we have seen, results in declining perceptual, cognitive, motivational and motor-related skills and competencies. Sleep, mood and health status, in turn, are reciprocally related. In short, sleep is something we cannot do without; sooner or later it 'catches up with us' so to speak[10].

This, however, leaves us little further forward when it comes to understanding some of the more sociological dimensions of sleep, the social construction of sleep considered in this chapter notwithstanding. Therefore it is to these very issues, set against the backdrop of these preliminary or provisional considerations of the nature and status of sleep, that we now turn in the remainder of the book, starting with an exploration of changing patterns and practices of sleep across the centuries.

Notes

1 It was also through the clinical insights of Constantin von Economo, and his pathological investigations of the brains of patients who had died, that the identity of *Encephalitis Lethargica* (sleepy-sickness) was established. See, for example, von Economo (1931). See also Chapter 5 in this book.

2 Nowadays of course, in the modern sleep lab, full polysomnogram recordings are usually taken, including the electroencephalogram (EEG), the electro-oculogram (EOG) to record eye movement and the electromyogram (EMG) to record electrical activity in muscles. Internationally agreed criteria for interpreting the polysomnogram were published in 1968 (Rechtschaffen and Kales 1968). See Morgan (1987: Ch. 1) for a useful account of the *measurement* of sleep in historical context.

3 Mention should also be made, at this point, of the 'nocturnal erection' during REM sleep: an erect penis, that is to say, for healthy men of all ages, and an engorged clitoris, lubricated vagina and erect nipples in females. A middle-aged man, for example, 'will typically have three or four full erections during the course of the night, each lasting about half an hour' (Martin 2003: 232). Their duration does decline with age, in line with the overall decline in sleep. Otherwise, the nocturnally erect penis remains 'remarkably unbowed with age' (2003: 132). Nocturnal erections, however, have little or nothing to do with sex or erotic dreams: they accompany REM *irrespective* of such factors. Perhaps most important of all, in the context of the present chapter, the first scientific account of this phenomena appeared in 1944. Thus, as Martin astutely comments, a 'scientific paper describing perhaps the most easily visible hallmark of REM sleep was published eight years before Eugene Aserinsky discovered REM sleep from his son's EEG traces' (2003: 133).

4 Morgan also draws attention here to Ralph Berger's (1961) finding, at the University of Edinburgh, of REM sleep-related muscle relaxation in human subjects: a finding which 'has further refined the ability of researchers to distinguish between REM and non-REM sleep' and has since warranted the inclusion of additional measurement of muscle (usually chin muscle) activity via the EMG, in combination with the EEG and the EOG, in most all-night recordings (Morgan 1987: 7) – see also note 2 above.

5 We know, for example, in evolutionary terms, that NREM sleep is older than REM sleep. The possible functions of sleep, moreover, include restorative/conservatory/building roles that are fitness enhancing and associated especially with NREM sleep, and information processing roles associated with REM sleep. Crick and Mitchison (1983, 1995), for instance, on this latter information processing count, put forward the 'reverse-learning theory' of REM sleep, which proposes that the biological function of REM sleep is to help avoid overloading the brain by getting rid of weaker, unwanted or unnecessary memory traces in favour of stronger ones: an effective and efficient form of memory housekeeping if you like, which sifts and sorts the wheat from the chaff. This, in turn, they argue, has helped evolution construct much smaller brain sizes than would otherwise have been necessary. The evidence for this hypothesis however, Martin (2003: 248) comments, is not altogether convincing. 'The mystery of sleep function', as Hobson (1995: 189) himself admits, 'is still impenetrable'.

6 Caution is needed here, given the retrospective nature of this account, which itself, moreover, is part of a broader debate on the nature and status of sleep apnoea as a clinical disorder, and the evolution of modern day 'sleep medicine' – see Chapter 5 for a fuller discussion of these issues.

7 Thanks to Jonathan Reinarz for drawing this source to my attention.

8 Thanks again to Jonathan Reinarz for this reference.

9 The terminology, to be sure, is hazardous here. Unfortunately, as Mavromatis (1987: 3) notes, there is no English equivalent to the Italian term 'dormiveglia' (sleep-waking) that captures, so succinctly, both 'hypnagogic' and 'hypnopompic' states: 'hypnagogia', nonetheless, is Mavromatis's own preferred collective term.

10 Yawning too, of course, is another great mystery that, rightly or wrongly, is associated with sleep. Explanations for this strange phenomenon (which is not simply confined to humans) abound, including the well known theory of a drop in blood oxygen levels (or a rise in blood carbon dioxide levels if you prefer); the theory that yawning aids the physiological development of the lungs in early life; and, the theory that yawning helps prepare us for a 'gear-change' in activity level. The limited scientific evidence to date on this matter tends to support the latter explanation, namely, that yawning has little or nothing to do with tiredness or boredom, but precedes and prepares us for a change of gear, whether physical, mental or both (Martin 2003: 138–41).

Chapter 2

Sleep through the centuries: historical patterns and practices

Introduction

It is one thing to document changing theories and explanations of sleep, quite another to trace or tap into changing patterns and practices of sleep across the centuries – a doubly difficult task in fact given that precious little has been written directly on these dormant matters by historians themselves. If sleep constitutes a third of our lives, then, one might say, a third of the past is missing from the history books. Thankfully, however, things are not quite as dire or as desperate as that. There are indeed many different sources we can turn to for direct and indirect glimpses or testimonies of sleep in the past, sources taken together that help us recover or reclaim the 'hidden history' of sleep. *When*, *how*, *where* and with *whom* did people sleep in the past? These are some of the questions this chapter seeks to address if not fully answer.

The focus, of necessity, is somewhat partial or selective, with a particular emphasis on re-reading key sociological sources, including the likes of Elias, Foucault and Weber, alongside other related works and insights on sleeping practices from the dim and distant past. First, however, a word from no greater source than the Bible itself: the genesis of many dormant visions and insights, both sacred and profane.

Let there be light: biblical bodies and dormant/dozy disciples. . .

In the beginning, we are told, God created heaven and earth. Earth was without form and void, and darkness was upon the face of the deep. And God said 'Let there be light: and there was light'. And God saw the light, and it was 'good', and God 'divided the light from the darkness', calling the light 'Day' and the darkness 'Night: And the evening and the morning were the first day'. God, in fact, made two great lights: the 'greater light' to rule the day, and the 'lesser light' to rule the night: he made the stars also (Genesis Ch. 1: verses 1–16). On the Seventh day of Creation God ended his work and he 'rested', blessing and sanctifying the Seventh day as the day of 'rest' (Genesis Ch. 2: verse 3). The seven-day week, conceived in these terms, has certainly stood the test of time, from Sumerian and Babylonian (pre-Biblical) civilizations to the present day, although the seventh day of 'rest' is now very much under attack, of course. The Romans, apparently, dabbled with an eight-day week, but thought better of it and reverted to seven (Martin 2003: 24).

Biblical references to sleep and rest extend far beyond God's creation of light and the advent of the seven-day week, to a range of other important themes and issues. Dreams, for example, are a prominent if not perennial theme in the Bible: the source of many great prophecies and revelations such as Jacob's ladder. Biblical dreams could also inspire hatred and envy. Joseph, for instance (the son of Jacob, who wore a splendid coat of many colours), dreamed a dream that spoke to him of reigning or ruling status. Upon reporting this dream to his jealous brethren, hatred ensued. Joseph, nonetheless, had another dream and said: 'Behold, I have dreamed a dream more; and, behold, the sun and the moon and the eleven stars made obeisance to me', upon which his own loving father rebuked him and his brethren envied him still more, conspiring against him (Genesis Ch. 37, verses 9 and 10).

As for biblical beds, the Hebrews it seems borrowed freely from the forms of their neighbouring nations, especially Egypt, during their long stay there (Wright 1962). A bed in the book of Proverbs, for example, is 'decked. . .with coverings of tapesty, with carved works, and with fine linen of Egypt' (Ch. 7, verse 16). But, Wright comments, once we have identified, from the many mentions of beds in the Old Testament, 'the few that are not merely incidental to its favourite themes of sloth, adultery, incest and murder', we are 'left with little information' (1962: 8). Apart from Lazarus in the New Testament, who was commanded to take up his bed and walk, moreover, we can note the 'odd fact that the Saviour, though he is born in a manger and is once found asleep in a boat, is never mentioned going to bed' (1962: 8).

This comment leads nicely to what is, perhaps, the most telling reference to sleep in the Bible; the betrayal of Christ, not simply by Judas but by his own dozy or dormant disciples. The scene in the Garden of Gethsemane is well known, but no less painful or instructive for that:

> And he cometh unto the disciples, and findeth them asleep, and said unto Peter, What, could ye not watch with me one hour?
>
> Watch and pray, that ye enter not into temptation: the spirit indeed is willing but the flesh is weak.
>
> He went away again the second time, and prayed. . .
>
> And he came and found them asleep again: for their eyes were heavy.

And he left them, and went away again, and prayed for a third time. . .

Then cometh unto his disciples and saith unto them, Sleep on now, and take your rest: behold, the hour is at hand, and the Son of Man is betrayed into the hands of sinners.

(St Matthew, Ch. 26, verses 40–5)

Enter Judas!

The implications of this passage hardly need spelling out. Nonetheless, in keeping with the foregoing themes, it does tell us much about Biblical attitudes to sleep: the spirit, to repeat, may be willing, but the flesh indeed is weak!

Civilized bodies

If biblical bodies provide one important starting point on the trail of sleep through the ages, then the Eliasian notion of 'civilized bodies' provides another; a more thoroughgoing sociological one at that. Elias's (1978/1939) work on the 'civilizing process' provides a rich source of insights into changing sleeping arrangements through the centuries, particularly the etiquette of the bedroom. The general thesis here, in keeping with the civilizing process in general, is that sleep has become an increasingly *private* matter, like all other 'natural' or 'animal' bodily functions. What is and is not said in manners books over the centuries, in this respect, is his prime source of data. On behaviour in the bedroom, for example, Erasmus' *De Civilitate Morum Puerilium* (1530) instructs his readers as follows:

If you share a bed with a comrade, lie quietly; do not toss with your body, for it can lay yourself bare or inconvenience your companion by pulling away the blankets.

By the eighteenth century, however, the reader of La Salle's (1774 edition) *les Regles de la bienseance et de la civilité chrétienne*, is told:

It is a strange abuse to make two people of different sex sleep in the same room. And if necessity demands it, you should make sure that the beds are apart, and that modesty does not suffer in any way from this commingling. Only extreme indigence can excuse this practice. . .

If you are forced to share a bed with a person of the same sex, which seldom happens, you should maintain a strict and vigilant modesty. . .

When you have awakened and had sufficient time to rest, you should get out of bed with fitting modesty and never stay in bed holding conversations or concerning yourself with other matters. . .nothing more clearly indicates indolence and frivolity; *the bed is intended for bodily rest and for nothing else.*

(Both quoted in Elias 1978/1939: 162–3, my emphasis)

Slowly but surely, Elias notes, the bedroom has become 'one of the most "private" and "intimate" areas of human life'. Sleep, in this respect, has 'shifted behind the scenes of social life' (1978/1939: 163). The nuclear family, he ventures, 'remains the only legitimate, socially sanctioned enclave for this and many other functions. Its visible and invisible walls withdraw the most "private", "intimate", irrepressibly "animal" aspects of human existence from the sight of others' (1978/1939: 163).

In medieval society, in contrast, this function had not been privatised or separated from the rest of social life. People often slept in daytime and in any place that was convenient. Sleeping, in other words, was a relatively 'public' undifferentiated matter, and the physical space in which it occurred was shared, not infrequently by many others: 'In the upper class, the master with his servants, the mistress with her maid or maids; in other classes, even men and women in the same room, and often guests staying over night' (1978/1939: 163). Sleep, in short, including the sleeping–waking cycle itself, was a relatively 'undisciplined', 'undifferentiated' affair at this time, not least as far as daytime sleep was concerned: anywhere, anytime, one might say.

In general, Elias continues, people 'slept naked in lay society', and in 'monastic orders either fully dressed or fully undressed according to the strictness of the rules' (1978/1939: 163). Gradually, however, this unconcern disappears, slowly in the sixteenth century and more rapidly in the seventeenth, eighteenth and nineteenth centuries; first in the upper classes and much more slowly in the lower classes. A special nightdress, for instance, came into being at roughly the same time as the fork and the handkerchief. Like the other 'implements of civilization', it is a symbol of:

> . . .the decisive change taking place at this time in human beings. Sensitivity to everything that came into contact with the body increased. Shame became attached to behaviour that had previously been free of such feelings.
>
> (Elias 1978/1939: 164)

A slight relaxing of these strictures seems to have occurred since the First World War. Sleep, Elias claims, is 'no longer so intimate or segregated as in preceding stages'. There are more situations in which people are exposed to the sight of strangers sleeping, undressing, or dressing[1]. As a result, nightclothes (like underwear) 'have been developed and transformed in such a way that the wearer need not be "ashamed" when seen in such situations by others' (1978/1939: 166).

The general thrust of the civilizing process clearly indicates how sleep, becoming slowly more 'intimate' and 'private', is 'separated from most other social relations', and how 'precepts given to children and young people take on a specific moralistic undertone with the advance of feelings of shame' (Elias 1978/1939: 166). Children indeed, Elias argues, 'necessarily touch again and again on the adult threshold of delicacy, and – since they are not yet adapted – they infringe the taboos of society, cross the adult shame frontiers, and perpetuate emotional danger zones which the adult himself [*sic*] can only control with difficulty' (1978/1939: 167). The changes taking place in manners books over the centuries, from this perspective, closely mirror those required in the life of each individual child in the process of growing up: what Elias terms the sociogenetic ground rule.

All in all then, in much the same way as eating, the 'wall between people', the 'reserve', the 'emotional barrier' erected by conditioning between one individual and another, grows continuously:

> To share a bed with people outside the family circle, with strangers, is made more and more embarrassing. Unless necessity dictates otherwise, it becomes unusual even within the family for each person not to have his (*sic*) own bed and finally – in the middle and upper classes – his own bedroom. . . . Only if we see how natural it seemed in the Middle Ages for strangers and for children and adults to share a bed can we appreciate what a *fundamental change in interpersonal relationships and behaviour is expressed in our manner of living*. And we recognise how *far from self-evident it is that bed and body should form such psychological danger zones as they do in the most recent phase of civilization* . . . .
>
> (1978/1939: 168, my emphases)

Despite these important insights, the picture Elias paints of sleep is both tantalisingly brief and partial, particularly as far as the lower ranks and segments of society are concerned (for further Eliasian commentaries on these dormant issues see Gleichman 1980 and Mennell 1989). Elias' analysis, indeed, begs as many questions as it answers. Did sleep, for example, routinely offer individuals genuine repose? Did most, in the era before modern day sleeping pills, pillows and the like, enjoy undisturbed rest? Did all social classes, moreover, enjoy sleep equally? Is sleep, to quote again Sir Philip Sidney's famous phrase, 'Th' indifferent judge between the high and the low'?

Answers to these and many other important questions are to be found in Ekirch's (2001) illuminating study of pre-industrial slumber in the British Isles. Again, echoing the sentiments of this book, Ekirch underlines the fact that historians, like sociologists, have tended to neglect sleep-related matters, including bedtime rituals, sleep deprivation and variations in slumber between different social ranks; an 'historical indifference' which Samuel Johnson lamented way back in the eighteenth century[2].

So how did people sleep, and did this vary according to social rank? The medieval notion of 'sleep of the just', Ekirch (2001: 346) comments, certainly suggests that soundest sleep belonged to those of lower social rank who toiled hard. Amongst leading authorities, moreover, a sound night's slumber was deemed critical for withered spirits, bodily health and increased longevity. Bed, in this respect, was 'medicine of a kind' (2001: 348; see also Chapter 1 in this book). Six to eight hours was a common reference point here as far as one's length of slumber was concerned, but this varied according to season and constitution or complexion. Dr Andrew Borde, for example, in his *Compendious Regiment, or Dietarie of Health* (1542), instructs us that 'Old ancient doctors of physic saith eight hours of sleep in summer and nine in winter is sufficient for any man; but I do think the sleep ought to be taken as the complexion of man is' (Borde 1542, quoted in Wright 1962: 194)[3].

In truth, however, Ekirch contends, the pre-industrial era was one in which few adults beneath the upper social ranks enjoyed the opportunity or luxury of sleeping more than seven or eight hours. Despite the Biblical injunction to rest at night-time, indeed, pre-industrial subsistence pressures and workplace demands deprived many folk of their sleep or slumber (2001: 348–50). Night-time, too, afforded households:

> . . .precious opportunities for sociability and leisure, which frequently accompanied spinning, mending, and other "evening workes" by the hearth. In villages, men frequented taverns and neighbors gathered within homes to enjoy the resonant talents of storytellers. Large towns and cities featured a growing array of nighttime diversions ranging from masquerades and assemblies to brothels and nighthouses.
>
> (2001: 350)

Diaries, in this respect, whilst heavily weighted toward the upper classes, suggest that adults retired to bed between 9 and 10 o'clock and typically slept for periods of six to eight hours (2001: 350).

Elaborate rituals were also followed as bedtime approached. Sleep, in these pre-modern times, was a period of unparalleled vulnerability, if not anxiety (2001: 353). This included not simply fears of nightmares and of nocturnal intrusions of various sorts, both real and imagined, but the nightly removal of pests, including fleas and bedbugs. As for the warming of beds on cold winter nights, devices ranged from warming pans for the better off, to hot stones wrapped in rags for those with fewer means at their disposal (Ekirch 2001; Wright 1962). Nightwear too, to repeat Elias' earlier observation, was a class-specific affair, with more elaborate regalia, including chemise and socks, adopted by the middle and upper classes by the sixteenth century, and other more 'coarse night gear' (at most), adopted by the lower classes. Frequently people slept naked or in their day clothes to save the expense of blankets and to save on time when rising in the morning (Ekirch 2001: 355).

Other bedtime rituals, Ekirch reports, included various bodily ablutions and hair combing practices, performed by servants for the well-to-do (Pepys' diary, for example, is a rich source here) not to mention the imbibing of laudanum – especially popular amongst the propertied classes – and the conducting of household prayer in order to set the mind at rest for the night ahead, bringing many comforts. In addition, less affluent households routinely invoked magic, including nightspells, the hanging of amulets, the reciting of charms to avert nightmares, and the use of potions to prevent bedwetting and to facilitate sleep (2001: 357).

Perhaps Ekirch's greatest insights into pre-industrial slumber, however, pertain to the very *nature* and *quality* of sleep at this time. In countering the wistful and romantic notion that the sleep of our ancestors or forebears was a tranquil affair of peaceful repose, from dusk to dawn, Ekirch seeks to expose a common myth of modern-day thinking. Far from this idyllic stereotype, he contends, early modern slumber remained a precarious affair in which intermittent disruptions abounded: 'much more so, in all likelihood, than does sleep today' (2001: 358). Despite the elaborate precautions listed above to ensure a sound night's sleep within households of all classes, many early references to sleep indeed:

> . . .contain such adjectives as "restless", "troubled", and "frightened". A seventeenth century religious devotion spoke of "terrors, sights, noises, dreams and paines, which afflict manie men" at rest. Exacting the greatest toll were physical maladies all the more severe after sunset, ranging from angina, gastric ulcers, and rheumatoid arthritis to such respiratory tract illnesses as asthma, influenza, and consumption (pulmonary tuberculosis). Making sleep all the more onerous, whatever the strain of sickness, is that sensitivity to pain intensifies at night.
>
> (2001: 358)

Dental pain, through decaying and rotten teeth, was also a common complaint at this time, which must have left its victims equally vulnerable to sleepless nights: a fact still very much in evidence in nineteenth-century dental hospital records, many of which mention patients' inability to sleep[4]. The 'pains of sleep' mentioned in Chapter 1, including those of Coleridge (1971, 1985), add further weight to these contentions. The *quality* of sleep, compared to later times, was far from guaranteed for our ancestors, rich or poor. The middle classes, to be sure, may have enjoyed more comfortable repose, but no class it seems could bank on a sound or silent night, given the manifold ills and interruptions it harboured. Pepys' (1993/1660–69) diary is instructive on this count. In his diary entry for September 3rd 1664, for example, Pepys reports a suspected case of nocturnal flea-biting, but is subsequently proved wrong:

> I have had a bad night's rest tonight, not sleeping well, as my wife observed, and once or twice she did wake me; and *I thought myself mightily to be bit with fleas, and in the morning she chid her maids for not looking the fleas a-day.* But when I rise, I find that is only the change of weather from hot to cold, which (as I was two winters ago) doth stop my pores, and so my blood tingles and itches all day over my body.
>
> (my emphasis)

Other physical hazards, however, appeared to stem from bedsharing itself:

> Waking this morning out of my sleep on a sudden, I did with my elbow hit my wife a great blow over her face and nose, which waked her with pain – at which I was sorry. And so to sleep again.
>
> (January 1st 1662).

As for the cold, Pepys' diary entry for December 14th 1661 states: 'All the morning at home, lying a bed with my wife – such a habitt we have got this winter, of lying long abed'.

To these observations, we may add Pepys' nocturnal fears for the safety of his house, which frequently kept him awake or prompted fitful slumber: 'The truth is', he tells us, 'my house is mighty dangerous having so many ways to be come to. . .God preserve us this night safe!'

This may well be so. The sleep of the working poor and the destitute, nonetheless, remained particularly vulnerable to the vicissitudes of everyday/everynight existence, including 'unwelcome intrusions, frigid temperatures, annoying noises, voracious insects, and the stench of nightsoil' (Ekirch 2001: 359). Again we return here to Eliasian observations concerning the sharing of sleeping spaces, beds and bedding – a practice that persisted for a considerable time amongst the lower ranks of society. 'To pig', for example, was a common practice and a well-used term in England in the pre-industrial era: sleeping, that is to say, with one or more bedfellows (Ekirch 2001: 361). Probably most parents slept apart from children other than infants, Ekirch contends, although occasionally *entire households* of European peasants shared the same bed. Some families, moreover, throughout the British Isles, brought farm animals within sleeping quarters at night, thereby serving a dual purpose: first, the protection of livestock from thieves and predators; second, the provision of warmth, albeit off-set by the nasty smell (2001: 361).

Far from blissful repose, ordinary folks probably suffered 'some degree of sleep deprivation, feeling more fatigued on awakening at dawn than retiring at bedtime' (Ekirch 2001: 362). Napping during the day, in this respect, was a common practice which had less to do, Ekirch argues, with the pre-industrial work ethic and more to do with poor quality of sleep and the consequent levels of fatigue that afflicted the early modern population (2001: 362). Ekirch goes one or more steps further here, pointing to an entirely different pattern of 'segmented slumber' at this time; one that has been overlooked or neglected in commentaries and debates on sleep ever since. Until the close of the early modern era, he contends, Western Europeans on most evenings experienced 'not one but two major intervals of sleep, bridged by up to an hour or more of quiet wakefulness' (2001: 364). Certainly there are plenty of sources and anecdotal accounts that bear witness to this custom and practice, from Homer through Shakespeare to Stevenson. The initial interval was usually referred to as 'the first sleep' or less often the 'first nap' or 'dead sleep', followed by an intervening period of consciousness or 'watching' (cf. Willis's 'Watching evil' in Chapter 1) and a succeeding interval of slumber called 'second' or 'morning sleep'. The later at night the individual went to bed, however, 'the later they stirred after their initial sleep; or, if they retired past midnight, they would likely not have awakened until dawn' (2001: 365). This practice, it seems, was taken-for-granted and hence required no elaboration; sleeping by 'interval', was common practice, if not the unspoken 'norm' right up to the dawn of the modern-day industrial era.

How are we to explain this curious anomaly, which, with the benefit of historical hindsight, has more to do with our own peculiar 'consolidated' sleep pattern today than the aberrant 'segmented' ways of our ancestors? The answer for Ekirch, drawing on the findings of modern day sleep science, concerns the introduction of artificial light which has had a 'profound effect' on our biological clocks and hence our current sleep patterns. Various studies, as noted in Chapter 1, have shown that modern people, when deprived of artificial light, revert to a 'basic' pattern of 'broken' sleep or 'segmented' slumber which mimics that of our pre-industrial counterparts (2001: 367–8).

This in turn begs another important question: what did our pre-industrial ancestors do with this intervening period of wakefulness, between first and second sleep? Some, apparently, lay quietly and simply reflected on events of the preceding day or contemplated the day to come. Others, however, rose from their bed for a variety of purposes, most often to urinate. Praying or conversing with one's bedfellow seems to have been a fairly common practice, as was the conduct of 'intimate relations'. Many children, Ekirch contends, were probably conceived in the night, at just this point in time. Awakenings in the dead of the night also, of course, provided ample opportunity for petty crime, from stealing in urban settings to pilfering in the countryside (2001: 370). Perhaps most significant of all, was the opportunity this segmented slumber provided for people to share or stay in touch with their dreams and associated hypnagogic states, providing a rich source of interpretation and storytelling. Had pre-industrial families not stirred until dawn, Ekirch speculates:

> . . .many of these visions of self-revelation, solace and spirituality would have perished by the bedside – some lost in the throes of sleep, others dissipated by the distractions of the day – 'flitting with returning light'. . . .
>
> (2001: 381)

This passing of segmented sleep did not, however, take place overnight. Beginning in 'the late seventeenth century, segmented sleep slowly but surely grew less common, first amongst the propertied classes in better-lit urban neighbourhoods, then among other social strata in all but the most cloistered communities' (2001: 383). Not until the early nineteenth century, however, would darkness be eroded in larger English localities through industrialisation and the steady growth of 'leisured affluence among urban and middle upper classes'. Professional policing, nocturnal trade, evening employment, improvements in domestic lighting and illumination of public places and streets, these and many other developments increasingly rendered 'night less obscure. . . . Hours once dominated by darkness grew more familiar' (2001: 383). As a consequence, segmented slumber was duly confined to the past.

The effect on sleep of modern forms of lighting, then, if this thesis is correct, has been truly immense. Our *quality* of sleep, in this respect, may well have improved over the centuries, but its *quantity* continues to diminish. But this is perhaps not the most significant factor in the balance sheet of gains and losses. What also weighs heavily in any such balance sheet is the fact that:

> . . .our assimilation of nocturnal visions has gradually waned, and with it, a better understanding of our deepest drives and emotions. If not the 'royal road' to the unconscious posited by Freud, dreams nonetheless afforded innumerable generations a well-travelled if winding path to self-awareness. It is no small irony that, by turning night into day, modern technology, while capable of exploring the inner sanctums of the brain, has also helped obstruct our oldest avenue to the human psyche. That, very likely, is the greatest loss, to paraphrase Thomas Middleton, of having been 'disanulled your first sleep, and cheated of our dreams and fantasies'.
>
> (Ekirch 2001: 385)

If Elias casts important light on the 'civilizing' or 'privatising' or 'sequestration' of sleeping bodies over the centuries, Ekirch enriches and emboldens the picture through a series of extraordinary insights into the 'segmented' slumber of pre-industrial times. Sleep, in short, may have been no idyll in the past, and the *quality* of our sleep may have grown appreciably since this time, but we may also have lost something vital in the process. . . .

Disciplined/ascetic bodies

Another way of looking at these issues comes through a close re-reading of the writings of Foucault and Weber. *The History of Sexuality, Vol 2* and *Vol 3* (Foucault 1987, 1988), for example, contain many important insights into sleep and dreams in Ancient Greek and Roman times, including Artemidorous of Daldis *Oneirocritica/The Interpretation of Dreams*. The analysis of dreams, Foucault reminds us, was one of the 'techniques of existence' at this time (see also Chapter 1 in this book).

The moral reflection of the Greeks around the fourth century BC, Foucault notes, was less concerned with interdictions of various kinds than with a certain stylised freedom that the '"free man" excercised in his actuality'. The main objective of this reflection, we are told, was to define the 'use of pleasure' in terms of a certain way of caring for one's body. The preoccupation, in this respect, was more 'dietic' than 'therapeutic': a matter of 'regimen aimed at regulating an activity that was recognised as being important for health' (1987: 97–8). Diet or regimen was a fundamental category through which human behaviour could be conceptualised at this time and it characterised the way in which one managed one's existence. Regimen, in other words, was a 'whole art of living', including:

> . . . exercises [*ponoi*], foods [*sitia*], drinks [*pota*], sleep [*hypnoi*] and sexual relations [*aphrodisia*], everything that needed to be 'measured'.
> (Foucault 1987: 101).

As an 'art of living', regimen in turn was a 'whole manner of forming oneself as a subject who had the proper, necessary and sufficient concern for his body: a concern that permeated everyday life, making the major or common activities of existence a matter both of health and ethics' (1987: 108). Sleep or *hypnoi*, it is clear, fits more or less readily into the picture here – an important part of regimen in this bygone era, and the origin no doubt of the very notion of sleep hygiene: a marriage, in effect, of *Hypnos* (god of sleep) and *Hugeia* (goddess of health).

What Foucault values most here it seems, in these Ancient Greek arts of living or existence and the uses of pleasure they spawned, is the fact that people at this time were free from the normalising pressures of modern-day life. They were, that is to say, able to exercise a certain 'liberty' or 'autonomy' of practice which sought to maximize pleasure, beauty and the power derived from life itself.[5]

These latter day concerns provide a striking contrast, if not a direct response or antidote, to Foucault's (1977) earlier preoccupations with disciplinary technologies of power/knowledge and the production of 'docile' bodies, traceable throughout European society from the late eighteenth century onwards. Again we can recover important sleep related themes and insights here too in Foucault's writings, not least concerning the spatial and temporal dimensions of the sleeping-waking cycle and the disciplining of docile if not dormant bodies.

From the organisation of architectural space to the temporal ordering of individuals through the timetable, the body, Foucault shows, became increasingly surrounded and invested by various techniques and technologies of power/knowledge that served to analyse, monitor, survey and fabricate it in useful, productive ways. Many disciplinary methods, of course, had long been in existence in monastries, armies and workshops. Nonetheless, the seventeenth and eighteenth centuries were a turning point as far as the history of such methods are concerned. These disciplines became 'general formulas of domination' – evident in prisons, schools, factories, barracks and hospitals – in which it was possible to control the individual's use of time and space hour by hour and transform them into docile yet productive or useful bodies in the very process of doing so. Thus, discipline produces 'subjected and practised bodies, "docile" bodies: increasing the forces of the body, in economic terms of utility, whilst diminishing these same forces, in political terms of obedience' (1977: 137–9).

In the first instance, Foucault notes, discipline proceeds from the distribution of *space*. In organising cells, places and ranks, the disciplines create complex spaces, including sleep quarters or 'dormitories', that at once are architectural, functional and hierarchical (1977: 148). The disciplines also, of course, through *timetables* and the control of activities, establish 'rhythms, impose particular occupations, regulate the cycles of repetition'. The disciplinary use of time, in this respect, differs from its traditional (monastic) form, which was essentially based on the principle of 'non-idleness': one in which wasting time was 'counted by God and paid for by men'. The main aim of the traditional timetable, in other words, was to 'eliminate the danger of wasting time – a moral offence and economic dishonesty'. Discipline, rather, arranges a far more positive economy:

> . . .it poses the principle of a theoretically ever-growing use of time: exhaustion rather than use; it is a question of extracting, from time, ever more available moments and, from each moment, ever more useful forces. This means that one must seek to intensify the use of the slightest moment, as if time, in its very fragmentation, were inexhaustible or as if, at least by an ever more detailed internal arrangement, one could tend toward an ideal point at which one maintained maximum speed and efficiency.
>
> (1977: 154)

The temporal problem then, for these disciplinary technologies of power/knowledge, was how one could 'capitalise' on the time of individuals and organise 'profitable durations'. The disciplines that analyse space, breaking up and rearranging activities, in other words, must also be understood in these terms as 'machinery for adding up and capitalising on time' (see also Thompson 1967)[6].

The *spatial* and *temporal* disciplining of sleeping as well as waking bodies is an important part of this nexus of power/knowledge. The prison, for example, is an 'exhaustive disciplinary apparatus' that assumes responsibility for all aspects of the individual, including physical training, aptitude to work, everyday conduct, moral attitude and state of mind (see also Chapter 4 in this book). The prison indeed, much more than the school, the workshop or the army (which all involve a certain 'specialisation'), is 'omnidisciplinary': an unceasing discipline that gives almost total power over the prisoner. Every aspect of the prisoner's life, including sleep, is subjected to these disciplines, conducted according to principles of *isolation* from everything that motivated the offence and the complicities that facilitated it. Work, alternating with meals, we are told, accompanies the convict to evening prayer, 'then a new sleep gives him an agreeable rest that is not disturbed by the phantoms of an unregulated imagination'. Work and isolation, in tandem, act as agents of 'carceral transformation' (Foucault 1977: 240–1).

From the monastery to the prison, the school to the military barracks, the hospital to the factory, then, Foucault charts the birth of a new disciplinary form of power/knowledge that renders bodies increasingly 'docile' and productive: a rationalisation, spatialisation and temporalisation of bodies, in effect, both sleeping and waking, according to new disciplinary mandates or imperatives of regulation and control from the eighteenth century onwards. This in turn, provides the underlying rationale for his later concerns, harking back to ancient Greek times, for ways of life and living free from these 'normalising' pressures and disciplinary technologies of power/knowledge: an ethics of existence and autonomy of practice in which pleasure, beauty and power derived from life itself are maximised.

There are, in fact, as various commentators have suggested, some interesting parallels if not convergences here between Foucault's early disciplinary treatment of these issues and Weber's classic analysis of the origins, nature and effects of rationalisation, not least his analysis of the (iron cage) of bureaucracy. Both Foucault and Weber, for example, see modern rational practices emerging from the monastery and the army and spreading outwards towards the factory, the hospital and the home (Turner 1992). Weber's iron cage metaphor may well be seen as '*anticipating* Foucault's concern for the impact of rational practices and discourses on the organisation of the body and populations in modern societies' (Turner 1992: 127–8). *The Protestant Ethic and the Spirit of Capitalism* (Weber

1974/1930), moreover, contains the 'core' of Weber's views on the origins, nature and effects of rationalisation, and the 'kernel' of his reflections on modernity and discipline. Protestantism, in this respect, generated a new form of 'possessive individualism' which legitimated the making of money and created a culture dedicated to hard work, asceticism and the transformation of the human environment (Turner 1992: 116).

Protestant writings at this time, Weber shows, were dominated by continual, passionately preached, virtues of hard work and unrelenting physical and mental labour in one's calling as the surest proof of genuine faith and spiritual salvation: a far cry, returning to Foucault, from the Ancient Greek 'arts of existence' or 'uses of pleasure'. Richard Baxter (1615–91), for instance, is an exemplar of the English strand of puritanism derived from Calvinism: views elaborated and expounded in his *Christian Directory* and *The Saints' Everlasting Rest*. Wasting time, Weber notes, is deemed the first, and in principle the deadliest, of sins within this puritan doctrine:

> Loss of time through sociability, idle talk, luxury, even *more sleep than is necessary for health, six to eight hours, is worthy of absolute moral condemnation*. It does not yet hold, with Franklin, that time is money, but the proposition is true in a certain spiritual sense. It is infinitely more valuable because every hour lost is lost to labour for the Glory of God.
>   (Weber 1974/1930: 157–8, my emphasis)

Accordingly, Baxter's principal work is dominated by the continually repeated virtues of hard continuous bodily or mental labour. *Labour* is, on the one hand, an 'approved *ascetic* technique', in sharp contrast not only to 'the Orient but to almost all monastic rules the world over'. It is, in particular, a safeguard or specific defence against all those temptations, including sexual temptations, which Puritanism united under the name of the 'unclean life'. Along with a 'moderate vegetable diet and cold baths', we are told, 'the same prescription is given for all sexual temptations as is used against religious doubts and a sense of moral unworthiness: "work hard in your calling"'. Unwillingness to work, in short, is 'symptomatic of the lack of grace' (Weber 1974/1930: 158–9).

This religious valuation of relentless hard work in a worldly calling served as the most 'powerful conceivable lever', in Weber's view, for the expansion of that attitude in life he termed the 'Spirit of Capitalism' (1974/1930: 172). Sleep, it seems, was one of the 'casualties' of this unholy alliance or elective affinity. Once capitalism developed, however, its prioritisation of formal rationality left little room for human feelings or sentiments. Capitalism, both past and present, requires the rational management of the body and emotions: if or when the latter are expressed, they are to be kept in the 'private spheres' of an individual's life or else put to work for commercial ends, *qua* the 'managed heart' (cf. Hochschild 1983, 1994).

This in turn, in Weber's view, contributed to the 'disenchantment' of the modern world as rationality infuses organisations, bureaucracies and the routinised structures of everyday life and living.

Benjamin Franklin (1706–90), in this respect, may well have embodied and exemplified the spirit of capitalism, where time is money, but it is Thomas Alva Edison (1847–1931), for our purposes, who quite literally sheds further light on these matters as far as sleep, or lack of it, is concerned. The archetypal American inventor, Edison took out over 1,000 patents in his lifetime, the first at the tender age of twenty-one. Edison by all accounts, in keeping with the aforementioned figures, harboured a somewhat negative view of sleep, or perhaps more correctly too much sleep, likening it to over-indulgence if not obesity. In 1920, for example, T.C. Martin, in his pamphlet *Edison at Seventy-Three*, wrote:

> Edison sleeps well at seventy-three. When he sleeps he does nothing else. . . . He seems to have the faculty of getting more rest out of two hours than most men get out of six or eight. A short-time ago he was working all around the twenty-four-hour clock, went to bed at half-past five one morning and was up at seven, having had about one and a half hours real sleep. When he went to breakfast he was asked, 'How do you feel this morning?' and he replied 'I would feel better if I had not overslept myself half an hour.'
>
> (quoted in Bryan 1926: 274)

As with many great people or geniuses Edison was, however, a famous napper; a principle he turned to his own advantage as a further aspect of his 'work'. Edison's strategy here, we are told, when reaching a sticking point in the creative process, was to take a 'cat nap' in which he would doze in his favourite armchair, holding steel balls in the palms of his hands. As he fell asleep, his arms would relax and lower, thereby letting the balls fall into pans on the floor. The noise would wake Edison up and very often he would emerge with an idea to continue the project (Bernd Jnr 1978, cited in Mavromatis 1987: 186).

This suggests that Edison made extensive use of 'hypnagogia' as a means of arriving at new ideas and inventions; a creative link one might say (Mavromatis 1987: 186–7). His inventions, though, have profoundly altered our sleep, not least the electric light bulb, as noted earlier. We may well have Edison to thank for many great inventions, including automatic telegraph systems, the mimeograph, the carbon microphone for telephones, the phonogram (precursor of the gramophone), even the industrial laboratory, but his legacy as far as sleep is concerned, is at best mixed and at worst disastrous: the beginning of the end, one might say, in a 24/7 world.

Blaming Edison is clearly too easy (or lazy) an option. Edison, like those before him, was very much a product of his time: a time, as Foucault and

Weber remind us, of unprecedented rationalisation in which time itself, quite literally, was 'capitalised' upon.

Reporting/reforming sleep: poverty, over-crowding and public health

In Chapter 1 it was suggested that the nineteenth century, in many respects, was the 'age of sleep theories'. It was also, however, as all good historians know, a time of many reports and reforms that provide us with yet another window on the regulation of sleep and sleeping in the past, particularly amongst the poor and the destitute. What we see here in fact is further evidence that the 'civilizing process', as Elias calls it, for material as much as social or cultural reasons, had not yet fully penetrated or incorporated the lower ranks of society, at least as far as sleeping arrangements or the etiquette of bodies and bedrooms are concerned.

Over-crowding, in fact, was still quite common at this time, particularly in Victorian slums and prisons, as reported by the likes of Henry Mayhew, George Godwin, James Kay and Thomas Beame[7]. The moral agenda here, Crook (2002) comments, was all too obvious, with dormant bodies depicted as being 'indiscreetly mixed', which in turn involved the transgression of important boundaries such as those between 'the married and the unmarried, the natural and the social, the male and the female, and the young and the old'. In this literature too, there is a clear association between 'the mingling of bodies, and drunkenness, indolence, criminality and disease: there is even, in some texts, the implication of incest' (Crook 2002: 2). A taboo, indeed, may well have surrounded the very mention of the word incest, but 'sanitary inspectors, medical officers of health, poor law guardians, school inspectors (truant officers), slum clergymen, were all, it seems, from their personal house-to-house visitations, prepared to state before official bodies, confidently and matter-of-factly, that incest existed' (Wohl 1976: 206).

A variety of interests and (moral) agendas, then, as this suggests, crystallised or coalesced around the living and sleeping conditions of the labouring population in general and the poor in particular in nineteenth century Britain. We see this very clearly, for example, in Edwin Chadwick's (1997/1842) *Report on the Sanitary Conditions of the Labouring Population of Great Britain*. A mixture of graphic detail, tragic descriptions, telling statistics and hard-hitting testimonies, the Report provided a 'well publicised analysis of the extent and scale of the problem of public health in Victorian Britain and a clear call to action' (Gladstone 1997). Eye-witness reports of the general conditions of residences of the labouring classes, for instance, include the testimony of Mr Harding, Medical Officer of the Epping Union, who states:

The state of some of the dwellings of the poor is most deplorable as it regards their health, and also in a moral point of view. . .in my opinion a great want of accommodation for bed-rooms often occurs, so that you may frequently find the father, mother and children all sleeping in the same apartment, and in some instances the children having attained the age of 16 or 17 years, and of both sexes; and if a death occurs in the house, and the person dies of the most contagious disease, they must either sleep in the same room, or take their repose in the room they live in, which most frequently has a stone or brick floor, which must be detrimental to health.

(Quoted in Chadwick 1997/1842: 14)

Even more horrendous conditions, if possible, are reported in lodging houses and lodging-shops. Chadwick, for example, cites the following evidence obtained from miners in Durham and Northumberland concerning the conditions in their lodging-shops – buildings erected by the proprietors of the mines for their workers to 'lodge' in. One miner, Williams Eddy, states:

Our lodging rooms were such as not to be fit for a swine to live in. In one house there was 16 bedsteads in the room upstairs, and 50 occupied these beds at the same time. We could not always get all in together, but we got in where we could. Often three at a time in bed, and one at the foot. I have several times had to get out of bed, and sit up all night to make room for my little brothers, who were there as washers.

Another workman, Joseph Eddy, states:

I consider the lodging-shops more injurious to the health of the miners than their work itself. So many sleeping in the same room, so many breaths, so much stour from their working-clothes, so much perspiration from the men themselves, it is impossible to be comfortable. Two miners occupy one bed, sometimes three. The beds are shaken once a-week on the Monday morning, when the miners come. Some miners make their beds every night. The rooms are in general very dirty, being never washed, and very seldom swept, not over once a-month. There is no ventilation, so the air is very close at night.

(Quoted in Chadwick 1997/1842: 111–12)

Whilst these lodging-shops, however appalling, accommodated labourers during the working week, other types of 'lodging houses', by the mid-nineteenth century, had acquired considerable reputations as 'places of vice', harbouring a motley ensemble of clientele, from thieves to prostitutes, beggars to ballad singers. These lodging houses, it is reported, not infrequently slept fifty or more people, in rat-infested rooms. Beds were said to be something of a rarity and all-night drinking, singing and card playing were common pastimes in these 'ragged dormitories' or 'houses of ill-repute' (Crook 2002: 4). There are echoes here, perhaps, of Rabelaisian medieval carnival culture, with its excessive/transgressive corporeal themes of 'degradation', 'inversion' and 'brimming' over-abundance (Bakhtin 1968)[8]. Systematic measures, therefore, were introduced to curb, reform and regulate these dens of iniquity from 1851 onwards, with the passing of Common Lodging Houses Act. By the end of the century most lodging houses were able to offer complete privacy and some, in fact, became quite 'austere institutions' (Crook 2002: 4).

All in all, what we have here is a sad and sorry tale of the living quarters and sleeping conditions of the lower ranks of Victorian society well into the nineteenth century. If we add to this the grim conditions of working life itself, in factories, mines and the like, and the hard physical toil and back-breaking labour it entailed (Engels 1999/1845, for example, accused the capitalists of 'social murder' of the working classes) one can only wonder at general levels of tiredness and fatigue at this time, to say nothing of the nature and quality of sleep itself: a point which echoes and amplifies Ekirch's (2001) earlier insights into pre-industrial slumber in the British Isles. Sleep may indeed be a welcome 'release' from these toils, but as Engels reminds us, other temptations (themselves the enemy of sleep) were ready to hand:

> The working man comes home from his work tired, exhausted, finds his home comfortless, damp, dirty and repulsive; he has urgent need for recreation, he *must* have something to make work worth his trouble, to make the prospect of the next day endurable. . . . His enfeebled frame, weakened by bad air and bad food, violently demands some external stimulus: his social need can be gratified only in the public house. . . . How can he expect to resist the temptation. It is morally and physically inevitable that, under such circumstances, a very large number of working men should fall prey to intemperance.
>
> (1999/1845: 113–14)

There is, however, one further (Foucauldian) dimension to these debates that links these moral and public health agendas to the calculation of precise respiratory 'norms' regarding the correct ratio of (sleeping) bodies to space. These very developments, Crook (2002) notes, built on the pioneering work of Antoine Lavoisier in the late eighteenth century, who first suggested not only that air was composed of two gases (oxygen and nitrogen) but that in closed spaces over a prolonged period of time the amount of oxygen in the air decreased and the amount of carbon dioxide increased. The remedy, Lavoisier concluded, was good ventilation and adequate space (see Duveen and Klickstein 1955 for a detailed account of Lavoisier's contribution to public health). These ideas were well received in Britain and throughout Europe and greatly elaborated during the nineteenth century, being steadily incorporated into the spatial dimensions of buildings during this period, including prisons, hospital, barracks and private dwellings. Respiratory norms, therefore, which themselves helped constitute the individual as a distinct or singular biological unit, prescribed the minimum amount of cubic space each individual was to enjoy whilst asleep (Crook 2002). This was a project for 'disciplinary institutions' such as prisons, hospitals and barracks, which dates in Victorian Britain from the 1840s onwards, including: the so-called 'separate system' in prisons, providing each inmate with their own cell containing privy accommodation, a wash basin, desk and foldable hammock (the minimum amount of space per cell, in the interests of health, being 800 cubic feet); and the so-called 'Nightingale system' in hospitals, which grouped beds into rectangular 'wards' leading off from a main corridor (the minimum volume of space per patient being 1,500 cubic feet). Soldiers too, following a Royal Commission Inquiry (1861) were now provided with their own beds in barracks – the precise number within a given barracks governed by the requirement each man be accorded a minimum of 600 cubic feet of space (Crook 2004). In this respect then, as Crook astutely observes, the reform or 'cellularisation' of sleeping bodies in these institutional sites and settings, at one and the same time embraced a complex array or admixture of sanitary, disciplinary and epistemological imperatives (Crook 2004: 3).

As for the domestic environment, notable developments from the 1850s onwards included the metal 'ticketing' of houses to show their total cubic space and the implementation of various bylaws to this effect (Crook 2002). The reform of domestic sleeping arrangements also included attempts by various housing associations to provide the poorer classes with (two or three) bedrooms. One of the first practical developments on this front, for example, was 'Prince Albert's Model Dwellings' of 1851 which comprised four flats in a block, with living-room, scullery, water-closet and three bedrooms, whose 'external ventilation' was thought worth mentioning (Wright 1962: 290–1). By the time of the Housing Act of 1935, indeed, the number of persons per dwelling was limited to: 1 room – 2 persons; 2 rooms – 3 persons; 3 rooms – 5 persons; 4 rooms – 7½ persons; 5 rooms – 10 persons (1962: 325). We should not forget, however, as Crook (2004: 7) rightly reminds us, that a great deal of working-class housing remained untouched: not until after the Second World War, in fact, did the Victorian slums finally disappear from our urban landscapes.

These developments in turn run parallel with other tracts and efforts specifically devoted to 'healthy' or 'hygienic' sleep measures and practices:

themes, as noted earlier, which date back to Ancient Greek and Late Renaissance times (see also Dannenfeldt 1986), receiving a further twist in the Victorian period and reaching their apex in the current late or post-modern climate (of which more in Chapter 6). The voice of the Ladies' Sanitary Association, for example, an upper-crust enterprise to reform the hygiene as well as the aesthetics of the bedroom, is to be heard at this time. In *The Bedroom and Boudoir* (1878), for instance, Lady Barker laments the fact that few rooms are built so as to remain thoroughly 'sweet, fresh and airy throughout the night' (quoted in Wright 1962: 297). Her recommendation, in this respect, was 'Tobin's Tube', which was four inches square and brought air from outside to a high point in the room, but she would not go so far as to risk the opening of the window overnight. Others, however, preferred 'O'Brien's Bed-Ventilating Tube' which fed air right into the bed. There was also 'Dr Arnott's Improved Ventilating Valve' in plain or ornamental form (Wright 1962: 297). As for the matter of beds, Lady Barker apparently preferred the 'new wire-spring mattress to the old frowtsy feather bed, which nevertheless long survives her day' (1962: 297).

To these 'sanitary' concerns we may add those of others, such as Dr W.W. Hall (1871), who, in his tellingly entitled *Sleep or the Hygiene of the Night*, instructs readers in the preface that:

> Between the closing of the chamber door at night and its opening in the morning, a third of human life passes away, and upon the manner of its employment the physical, mental and moral character of man [*sic*] largely depends.

If impure air is breathed in during this time, we are told, bodily disease and premature death will inevitably result. If improper habits are cultivated, moral contamination and physical deterioration will follow. If by these or other means sound and proper sleep is prevented, 'the mind sooner or later fails of its elasticity, its vigor and its life' to be followed by 'nervousness, weakness of the intellect, softening of the brain, insanity and death'. The pages that follow, therefore, were intended to urge the:

> . . . practical and individual application of these truths on the part of husbands, wives and children; hence every intelligent reader has a personal interest in ascertaining the most healthful method of filling up a portion of his [*sic*] existence which has such important bearings – in acquainting himself with
> 'THE HYGIENE OF THE NIGHT'. (Hall 1871: Preface)

An early twentieth century text, likewise, echoes and amplifies these sentiments. The hygiene of sleep, we are told, is surely only a matter of 'ordinary common sense'. In the first place:

. . . no one of whatever age ought to sleep in a room not ventilated as well as or better than the so-called 'living room' (as though one did not also live in a bedroom!). It is an axiom in personal hygiene that no one should sleep in air which has not some communication with the outer air.

(Harris 1910: 15)

As for the hours devoted to sleep, Harris comments, this is a very important matter, especially for children and young people. The opinion, we are told, is 'rapidly growing that the hours of sleep of the young at school might in many cases be lengthened and that no work, especially mental, should be done before breakfast'. The length of time passed in sleep, nonetheless, should 'never be fixed arbitrarily, but made to suit the constitutions of the persons concerned' (1910: 16): an echo, it seems, of Borde's previously quoted advice way back in the sixteenth century. These and many other factors – from the soporific effects of warm baths, massage and warm milk, to the elimination of unnecessary noise and the position of the head – weigh heavily in the balance sheet as far as sleep hygiene or the hygiene of the night are concerned (see also Jacobson 1938).

The nineteenth century reporting and reforming of sleeping or incestuous bodies, then, was a class-related affair: a moral as well as a public health agenda, which quite literally incorporated respiratory norms and hygienic measures into the very spatial dimensions of buildings if not the practices of their inhabitants. What we see here, in fact, on closer inspection, is an incredible array or admixture of ideas and practices, policies and principles, concerning *inter alia*: the body, its boundaries and its 'normal' respiratory needs, the 'reformatory agency and utility of space', the 'primacy of the nuclear family', and the 'social as a manageable locus of an all-encompassing set of moral forces and relations' (Crook 2004: 1). The spatial ordering of sleep and sleeping bodies, in short, was a multifaceted project embracing 'all manner of concepts and convictions. . .which lay at the very heart of the Victorian governmental imagination' (2004: 1).

Embedding history

Already we have glimpsed many historical references to *beds* of the past in the foregoing pages of this chapter. Beds, to be sure, cannot be equated with sleep, nor even the partaking of rest: we can be quite active, if not amorous, in bed. Beds do, nonetheless, reveal much about society's attitudes toward sleep, both past and present. It may, therefore, be worth elaborating a little further on the history of the bed at this point in the proceedings: the embedding of history one might say. Wright (1962) for example, in *Warm and Snug*, provides us with just such a history, from the bed of Cleopatra to Roman repose, biblical beds to Byzantine beds, not to mention bedtime in space. 'The history of the bed', he proclaims, in keeping with the foregoing themes, is 'interwoven with the histories of social, sexual and sanitary attitudes, of architecture and building, of interior decoration and furniture' (1962: viii).

The ancient Egyptians, Greeks and Romans, by all accounts, took their beds seriously. Egyptian beds, for example, were often elegant affairs reflecting high standards of craftsmanship. There seems to have been no real distinction between the day couch and the night bed at this time (Martin 2003). There was usually a foot panel to the bed, but no head panel because there were no pillows. Beds, moreover, for the wealthy and privileged, were often taken to the tomb: itself telling testimony to the Egyptian belief in death as merely a (slumbering) transition point between life and the afterlife (Martin 2003). Perhaps the most well known case in point, of course, is the tomb of King Tutankhamen (c. 1350BC). This spectacular archaeological find included a rich treasure trove of beds, from those made of ivory to great gilt couches, the sides carved in the shapes of elongated animals (such as lions, cows, hippopotami or crocodiles), with head-rests of lapis lazuli, faience or ivory (Wright 1962: 4).

Beds in ancient Greece were more like wooden couches, elaborately decorated or otherwise, upon which the Greeks would lie to eat. The Greeks, by all accounts, led a somewhat 'austere' home life as far as beds and bedroom furniture was concerned. Fine furniture was chiefly made for temples and other public buildings. A bedroom, consequently, would typically hold little more than a bed and perhaps a few coffers and light chairs (Wright 1962: 10). As for the bed-going of Spartan soldiers, this, we are told, was subject to Spartan rules which included the sharing of one tent by fifteen men until the age of thirty, and provision for soldiers to 'sleep out' if married, but only after the age of thirty, as a full citizen (1962: 10).

The Romans, whilst learning many of their ways from Greece, including Grecian simplicity in their home life, had further 'designs' on beds. Roman writings, Wright comments, never mention two or more beds in one room, except in over-crowded apartment blocks. Most beds, it seems, were single (*lectuli*); however, as well as ceremonial marriage beds, there were ordinary double beds (*lecti geniales*). Roman beds were constructed from a range of materials, some more precious than others, according to one's means:

> Wooden beds were of oak, maple, cedar, terebinth or *arbour vitae*. Some, of inferior wood, had imitation grain, or fine figured veneers. Others were inlaid with tortoise-shell, silver or gold; some were cast in bronze. Petronius describes the millionaire Trimalchio's bed as being of solid silver. Some had bronze feet with a wooden frame; others ivory feet with a bronze frame. The under-mattress was still woven of webbing or cord. On this went a stuffed mattress (*torus*) and a bolster, both filled according to one's purse with straw, reeds, herbs, wool, feather or swan down. Between the next two coverings the sleeper lay, and finally

there was a counterpane (*lodix*) or a gay damask quilt (*polymitum*). Canopies, curtains and mosquito nets were sometimes fitted. Roman beds would not be wholly comfortable by modern standards, but they could look quite impressive.

(1962: 12)

As for bedtimes, the habit in Roman times was to 'rise at dawn, and even those who lay in late might start the day's work in bed by the light of a candle or *lucubrum*, hence the word lucubration' (Wright 1962: 12). Getting up was a simple matter thanks to their bedtime attire. The Romans did not apparently strip at bedtime, save for the toga and sandals: undergarments were kept on day and night. Roman living, this suggests, was not necessarily luxurious.

For all centuries between the breakup or breakdown of the ancient empires and the reawakening of the Renaissance, household comfort, Wright assures us, hardly developed at all: 'the Ptolemies were as well bedded as the Plantagenets' (1962: 14). Northern European beds, in fact, remained fairly primitive devices until much more recently, save perhaps the beds of royalty or the rich. The latter, indeed, could be elaborate or luxurious affairs, with grand designs, fine bed heads, canopies and draperies, and sometimes satin sheets: something which reached its apex in the Tudor and Stuart periods (Martin 2003). Again we return here to the notion of beds as status symbols or a mark of distinction, the more elaborate and ornate, luxurious if not ludicrous, the better! Audiences in bed, for many of life's great events such as births, marriages and deaths, were customary. The bed-chamber, consequently, had to be furnished accordingly.

Nevertheless, we have seen that for the majority of plain, ordinary, everyday folk 'beds' could be as crude and as basic as bags of straw, hence the term 'to make a bed' in Saxon times, with whole families sleeping together on the floor (Martin 2003, Wright 1962). Between the fifteenth and seventeenth centuries English beds evolved from 'straw pallets on bare floors, to wooden frames complete with pillows, sheets, blankets, coverlets, and "flock mattresses", which were typically filled with rags and stray pieces of wool' (Ekirch 2001: 353). Wealthy households, in contrast, enjoyed elevated bedsteads, fine feather mattresses, and heavy curtains to prevent drafts and protect privacy (2001: 353). Already, it seems, families were investing in superior quality beds and bedding both for comfort and as a symbol of social prestige. Beds, Ekirch notes, were amongst the first possessions purchased by newly-weds as well as the first items bequeathed in wills. In modest homes, beds often represented 'over one-quarter of the value of all domestic assets, while for humble families, the bed was the piece of furniture first acquired on entering the "world of goods"' (2001: 352). People, as previously noted, were not the only occupants or incumbents of their beds, however. Bedbugs were a major hazard until the advent in the late eighteenth century of cheap cotton bedclothes, which could be boiled, and metal bedsteads, which provided no safe haven for these pests of the night (Ekirch 2001; Martin 2003).

As for the daytime nap or siesta, this was catered for during the seventeenth century through the advent of the *lit de repos*: a device created with the leisured classes very much in mind. Moliere apparently owned one hundred day beds, whilst a Versailles inventory lists forty-eight day beds of Louis XIV, some over seven feet long and up to three feet wide (Martin 2003; Wright 1962). King Louis indeed was somewhat obsessive when it came to ownership of beds, amassing an amazing total of 413 beds, of at least twenty-five varieties, including the *lit d'ange, á balaquin, á la dauphine, á la duchesse, á imperiale, en tombeau* and the *á la turque* (Wright 1962: 103).

The quest for grand or extravagant beds, however, gradually fizzled out in the early nineteenth century with the advent of the industrial revolution in which 'functional simplicity' reigned supreme, including iron or brass bedsteads and the introduction of the spring mattress in the 1850s (Martin 2003). All that remained it seemed, echoing previous themes, was to tackle the dreadful problem of overcrowding and the mingling of sleeping (if not incestuous) bodies amongst the urban poor and the destitute. Care of beds, bedding and bedrooms, moreover, was increasingly apparent, with many weird and wonderful devices to boot, particularly in (upper) middle class Edwardian households. A turn of the century publication by H.C. Davidson (1900), for example, entitled *The Book of the Home: A Practical Guide to Household Management*, has the following advice to give on servants and their duties:

> Having washed the front door-steps and polished the knocker and handle. . .the housemaid proceeds to the bedrooms, throws open the windows, and airs the beds; after which she makes them and arranges the bedrooms one by one.

Airing beds and bedding, we are told:

> . . .is most important, and should be thoroughly performed every day. The beds must be stripped of all clothing, which should be thrown back across a couple of chairs or over the rail at the foot of the bed, care being taken that the sheets do not drag on the floor. Mattresses, bolster, and pillows must be shaken and beaten, and any lumps among the stuffing dispersed; and *mattresses should also be turned up and brushed with a bed-whisk and 'button'-brush*, and if any feathers are escaping from any part of the bedding they should be pushed back and the seam of the tick sewn up.
>
> (1990: 220, my emphasis)

Bedroom windows, in turn, should be opened at the bottom and the top, as bad and heated air rises and passes out at the top, whilst cool fresh air comes in at the bottom. Windows, it is recommended, should remain open for a couple of hours each day, and for 'thorough ventilation' the door should be open as well.

As for 'travelling' beds of those 'on the move', the first such device was the man-powered, enclosed litter, with carrying handles for porters. People also slept in coaches, whilst beds for an important personage or invalid could be made up if sufficient room allowed (Wright 1962). The height of cosy coach-sleep, however, was reached in the field carriage used by Napolean in the campaign of 1815, a model of compactness which held a light bedstead of steel (1962: 261). The hammock too, of course, is an age-old device or invention, though not solely or simply for seafarers. A hammock, for example, was sometimes slung inside a coach. The first railroad 'sleepers' were introduced in the nineteenth century. George M. Pullman built the first US sleeping cars for the Bloomington–Chicago run on the Chicago and Alton Railroad in 1858. The first British sleeper, trailing somewhat behind so to speak, was built by the North British works at Cowlairs in 1873, with 'two three-berth compartments with three longitudinal berths in each, as well as servants' and a luggage compartment' (1962: 270). Passengers, we are told, had to bring their own bedding, and pay a supplement of 10 shillings over the first-class fare. Pullman sleepers were also imported the following year by the Midland Railway: a sign of things to come as far as British rail travel was concerned. Queen Victoria's two coaches for continental travel in the 'nineties, nonetheless, trumped all of this, containing 'a fine drawing-room, a dressing-room in Japanese style, and a bedroom with two beds, the larger for the Queen' (1962: 273). These and many other ways of sleeping 'on' or 'through' one's travels, whether by land, sea or air, attest not simply to human ingenuity and inventiveness but to our inescapable need to 'lie down' if not 'bed down' in some shape sense or form, whoever and wherever we are[9].

Beds today may be more or less elaborate affairs compared to the past, but either way they are surely more *comfortable*. A recent brochure from a leading British bed company, for example, boasts a variety of beds, classic or contemporary, single or double, fabric, metal or wood, not to mention the sofabed, all of which are designed to 'enrich your sleep life with luxury and style' (see also Chapter 5 in this book). Mattresses too have come on leaps and bounds, including a choice of open coil, pocket sprung, contour or latex. Perhaps most interesting of all, however, returning to the theme of beds in space, is the TEMPUR mattress: a self-proclaimed 'technological revolution in your bedroom'. The core of TEMPUR, we are told, is a high-tech visco elastic material, originally developed by NASA in the 1970s to protect and offer comfort cushioning for astronauts travelling in space. The TEMPUR material absorbs pressure at both heavy and light loads, and moulds to the shape of the body, giving a space-like feeling of 'weightless', which, in turn, its designers claim, is changing the lives of millions throughout the world by improving the quality their sleep lives.

Beds then, to summarise, comfortable or not, have proved an important historical reference point in people's lives, both past and present, stationary or on the move. They have also, of course, been the source of great inspiration over the centuries. Cicero and Pepys, for example, both wrote in bed, Rosini composed in bed, Proust and Mann loved their beds, and Churchill did much of his (morning) politicking in bed (Martin 2003). The bed, Guy de Maupassant states, 'is the symbol of life'. Are not 'some of our best moments spent in sleep?' But then again, 'we suffer in bed. It is the refuge of those who are ill and suffering; a place of repose and comfort for worn-out bodies, in one word, a part and parcel of humanity' (nd: 680–2). Embodiment and embedment, in short, are intimately related: a fact that historians, like sociologists, neglect at their peril. And so to bed, as Pepys would say. . .

Night as frontier?

A number of references throughout the discussion so far have been made to the historical relations between sleep and night-time if not darkness. Night-time, to be sure, may (still) be the most favoured time to sleep, but behind this 'truth' lies another rich story of nocturnal themes and issues worthy of amplification and elaboration in this final section of the chapter. Here we encounter the flip side, if flip side it is, of the arguments presented so far: a focus, that is to say, on the *active* uptake and transformation of night-time itself. To the 'doing' of sleep, to put it slightly differently, we might profitably add the 'doing' of night-time, or perhaps more correctly, its 'undoing'. The night, Alvarez (1996) notes, has many faces, including the literal and the metaphorical night, the dark of the moon and the dark of the night soul. Night-time, moreover, has been illuminated, negotiated, inhabited, feared, fancied, embraced and even ignored across the centuries, from the first (primitive) attempts to harness fire way back in the dim and distant past, to the modern day incandescent age. Nonetheless, however brightly or brilliantly we illuminate the night, Alvarez warns, 'the moral problem of the darkness won't go away' (1996: xiv). Nor, if we think of Edward Hopper's paintings, will the problems of loneliness and alienation.

There are, as this suggests, many fruitful lines of inquiry to pursue here. Like sleep, one may lament the paucity of sociological research on the 'dark side of life'. Night-time, one might say, has proved something of a 'black hole' compared to the sociology of everyday life (see also Steger and Brunt's 2003 critique of 'diecentricism')[10]. Let me, however, in this closing section of the chapter, focus on what, succinctly stated, amounts to the 'conquest' of 'outer darkness', if not the illumination of 'inner darkness'. We have,

Alvarez claims, in the last one hundred years or so, 'lost touch with the night'. 'True darkness', he contends, is a 'different order of experience and for twenty-first century man, who can eliminate it with the flick of a switch, it is mostly a source of pure terror' (1996: 3).

This may or may not be so, but whatever feelings greet darkness, night-time, sociologically speaking, has been something of a 'frontier' as far as the history of humanity is concerned. Melbin (1978, 1989), for example, takes up this thesis through a series of illuminating sociological observations which trade on these space–time relations and analogies. Humans, he wagers, are showing a trend toward more and more wakeful around-the-clock activity at all hours of the day and night. Large numbers of people are involved, and the trend is worldwide or global. Night, in this respect, may be seen as a 'frontier', and the 'expansion' into the dark hours may be seen as a 'continuation' of the geographical migration across the face of the earth. Social life in the night-time, he contends, has many important characteristics that resemble life on land frontiers (1978: 3). The subtext of Melbin's thesis, as this suggests, is a series of deliberations on the incessant (*qua* continuously wakeful, non-stop) society.

People, as already noted, have never solely or simply confined their activities to the daylight hours. Night-time has always had its 'ups' as well as its 'downs'. Around-the-clock activity though, as Melbin rightly contends, was only a small part of the whole or normal round of day-to-day life, until the nineteenth century. The pace and scope of wakefulness at all hours, in other words, has picked up appreciably from this point onwards, thanks in no small part to new means of artificial light – first, Murdoch's coal-gas illu-mination in the early nineteenth century, then Swan and Edison's electric light from the late nineteenth century onwards – and the ineluctable logic of capitalist accumulation and expansion: an expansion, to repeat, in both time (through the introduction of multiple shift-work) and space. In January 1882, when someone threw the switch for the first street lamps that used Swan and Edison's great invention, our perception of the world changed (Alvarez 1996: 19)[11]. On a darker note, the exploitation of human labour took a new turn at this time, as Marx himself commented (Melbin 1978: 4). Herein lies a trend that continues to the present day: an incessant or unremitting one at that. Today:

> More people than ever are active outside their homes at all hours, engaged in all sorts of activites. There are all-night supermarkets, bowl-ing alleys, department stores, restaurants, cinemas, auto-repair shops, taxi services, bus and airline terminals, radio and television broadcast-ing, rent-a-car agencies, gasoline stations. There are continuous-process refining plants, and three-shift factories, post offices, newspaper offices, hotels and hospitals. There is unremitting provision of some facilities – electric supply, staffed turnpike toll booths, police patrolling

> and telephone service. There are many emergency and repair services on-call: fire fighters, auto towing, locksmiths, suppliers of clean diapers, ambulances, bail bondsmen, insect exterminators, television repairers, plate glass installers and funeral homes.
>
> (Melbin 1978: 5)

Perhaps most interesting, for our purposes, is the question of how people behave at night-time? Does night-time, in other words, necessitate or result in different ways of acting or interacting? Night, for example, may well be a time of increasing fear, vulnerability and vigilance, given our diminished powers of visibility; a positive asset for those who choose to lurk in the shadows ready to pounce with malicious intent. This, in turn, places a question mark over the Goffmanesque 'civil inattention' accorded to others in the course of ordinary every*day* life. Active or excessive users of the night, moreover, are not only at risk through robbery and the like, they may also be cast as 'odd', 'eccentric', 'maverick' or 'deviant' by those whose inclinations are more in tune with daytime 'waking' hours. Melbin (1978, 1989), however, reaches some surprising conclusions here. When, and only when, it can be established that other users of the night are to be trusted, bona fide participants in these nocturnal dramas, then feelings of closeness, solidarity and comraderie quickly follow – feelings that are likely to be stronger than those engendered during the daytime and may even lead to the formation of new interest groups. More helpfulness and friendliness, indeed, is not uncommon; a contention Melbin backs up with some hard empirical evidence based on a variety of tests and experiments.

It is not simply, however, returning to the likes of Alvarez (1996), a question of the conquest or decline of 'outer' darkness, but the gradual illumination of 'inner' darkness, whether through recourse to the psychoanalyst's couch or the latest technological equipment of the sleep lab, not to mention the CT, MRI or PET scan.

The argument then is a simple yet sociologically illuminating one. Night-time or 'outer' darkness may well be a 'frontier', of sorts, which has steadily been conquered or colonised over the past century or so: an unrelenting or unremitting trend of incessant (wakeful) activity, which itself harbours a mixed bag of positives and negatives, depending on your point of view (see also Chapters 4 and 5 in this book). These similarities between the colonisation of space and time, however, as Melbin (1978: 21) himself acknowledges, cannot and should not be pushed too far. We should also, in other words, consider the 'uniqueness' of this 'new frontier', not least that 'expansion into the night can only go as far as the dawn'. The (rich) rewards for colonising land may be of a different order and kind to those of colonising the night: many people who work the night shift, for instance, are poorly paid with little or no decision-making latitude compared to their daytime counterparts. We can build upwards and outwards, but time, to all intents and purposes, is 'unstretchable' and 'unstorable'; we cannot 'save unused hours every night for further need' (Melbin 1978: 21).

Conclusions

Taking as our point of departure the changing nature of sleep or sleeping practices through the centuries, a variety of differing angles or vantage points have been considered in this chapter, each providing a window on sleep's 'hidden' past or history. This includes a recovery of sleep-related themes and issues through recourse to the Eliasian notion of 'civilized bodies' across the public–private divide, Foucauldian and Weberian insights into 'disciplined/ascetic bodies', and further glimpses into the unenviable lot of working-class, poor and destitute bodies in Victorian times, where themes of over-crowding and incest loom large through a mass of reports and reforms. Sleep, as this suggests, is no mere biological given, but an histori-cally variable phenomenon; an important indicator or index, in fact, of social order and social change. The spatialisation of dormant (working-class) bod-ies in the eighteenth and nineteenth centuries is particularly revealing on this count; a project of reform comprising or encompassing a complex admixture of sanitary, disciplinary and epistemological imperatives (cf. Crook 2002, 2004).

Embedded within all this, as we have seen, are further important insights into the 'sleep we have lost' in the transition to our incandescent if not incessant age. The conquest or decline of 'outer' darkness, in this respect, may well have been accompanied by the gradual illumination of 'inner darkness', thanks to the likes of psychoanalysis and the modern-day sleep lab, but at what cost? Whilst the *quality* of our sleep time, moreover, may well have improved over time, its *quantity* continues to decline. An unhappy note to end on, perhaps, but one we shall return to and further interrogate in Chapters 4 and 5.

Notes

1 One might see this as another manifestation or early indication of informalising trends. See Wouters (1986, 1987) on this latter Eliasian concept.
2 'Among the innumerable mortifications that waylay human arrogance on every side may well be reckoned our ignorance of the most common objects and effects', Johnson wagers. 'Sleep', he continues, 'is a state in which a great part of every life is passed'. Yet of this 'change so frequent, so great, so general, and so necessary, no searcher has yet found either the efficient or final cause; or can tell by what power the mind and body are thus chained down in irresistible stupe-faction; or what benefits the animal receives from this alternate suspension of its activities and powers' (Johnson 2003/1739–61: *The Idler*, No 32, Saturday, 25 November 1758).
3 Sources are many and varied here. Thomas Dekker, for example, who likened sleep to a 'delicate ambrosia', advised 'Sleep in the name of Morpheus your belly

full', the corollary being to sleep 'till your belly grumble' (Dekker, *The Guls-Horne-Booke* [1969/1609]). Samuel Johnson, in contrast, thought seven to nine hours a sufficient quantity. Old adages, moreover, abound and contradict one another. On the one hand, for instance, the saying goes: 'Six for a man, seven for a woman, eight for a fool'. On the other hand it is said that 'Nature requires five, Custom takes seven, Laziness nine, and Wickedness eleven' (quoted in Wright 1962: 194–5).

4 Dental hospital records. Samuel Adams Parker's (1862) *Remarks upon Artificial Teeth*, for example, records the case of a woman with decaying teeth, who was unable to sleep without resorting to 'strong narcotics'. Many others, nonetheless, could not resort to this luxury, probably turning to other alcoholic means to 'numb the pain'. A year later, in 1863, Adams Parker presented the details of four particularly interesting cases in the *British Journal of Dental Science*. Each one refers to patients suffering interrupted sleep, in one case for a period of seven years, others for two years, most for many months. Other patients at other hospitals probably suffered in much the same way, but no other published materials go into quite this sort of detail concerning disturbed sleep. I am grateful to Jonathan Reinarz for drawing this material to my attention.

5 Whilst *The History of Sexuality Vol 2: The Use of Pleasure* (Foucault 1987) is devoted to the manner in which sexual activity was 'problematised' in Classical Greek culture of the fourth century BC, *Vol 3: The Care of the Self* (Foucault 1988) deals with the same problematisation in Greek and Latin texts of the first two centuries AD. In doing so Foucault reveals, in the transition from the classical version of sexual pleasure to the golden age of the Roman Empire, an increasing *mistrust* of pleasure and a growing anxiety over sexual activity and its consequences.

6 E.P. Thompson's (1967) approach to time, work, discipline and industrial capitalism, of course, both complements and contrasts with Foucault's and Weber's treatment of these issues given its more Marxist leanings.

7 See Mayhew's (1851) *London Labour and the London Poor* (Mayhew nd.), for instance. See also Dyos (1967) on the slums of Victorian London.

8 Thanks to Chris Shilling for drawing this connection to my attention. See also Chapter 3 on the relationship between sleep, sexuality and intimacy.

9 One of the latest developments on the travelling beds front – a theme as pertinent to Chapter 4 as Chapter 2 – concerns British Airways' 'fully flat beds', measuring six feet (183 cm), introduced on the Club World Service. All you need to do, the would-be trans-Atlantic traveller is told, is 'lie back and relax into the fully flat bed, with even larger pillows and thicker blankets with luxurious double-sided cotton'. The cabin crew will even dim the lights, soon after take-off, to reduce nighttime disturbance, so that 'you'll not only get to sleep sooner, you can sleep longer, leaving you properly rested and energised for your day ahead' (www.britishairways.com/travel/sleeptrial/public/en_gb).

10 The charge of diecentrism in the social and cultural sciences alerts us to the manner in which daytime is apparently taken to be the standard for human existence with little or no attention to what takes place beyond daytime; a case of 'night blindness' in other words (Steger and Brunt 2003: 5; see also Brunt 2003; 2004).

11 See O'Dea (1958) for a social history of lighting dating back to the first sparks of illumination and the fire-making activities of our ancient ancestors.

Chapter 3

Sleep, embodiment and the lifeworld (*Lebenswelt*)

Introduction

It is now time, set against the backdrop of the preceding two chapters on changing theories and ideas, patterns and practices of sleep through the centuries, to examine more closely and intimately the relationship between sleep, embodiment and the lifeworld. The aim, in doing so, is to put further flesh on the bones of the arguments developed thus far, starting with a phenomenological investigation of the 'dormant' or 'sleeping' body, and moving outwards, so to speak, to other embodied themes and sociological issues concerning the 'doing' of sleeping across the life course, co-sleeping practices, and finally the literal and metaphorical links between sleep, death and dying. The chapter, in this respect, adds further phenomenological and sociological insights into sleep, which themselves provide a crucial bridge or stepping stone to broader sociological themes and issues taken up and addressed in the remaining two chapters: the 'missing link' one might say between the micro and macro domains.

What then of the dormant or sleeping body? Does sleep require or necessitate a rethinking of our previous notions of lived (waking or wakeful) embodiment? What, moreover, of related phenomenological states such as sleepiness or drowsy bodies? Where does this lead or leave us?

Falling/being 'asleep': phenomenological explorations

> . . .*we are not condemned to sustained flights of being, but are constantly refreshed by little holidays from ourselves. . .We are intermittent creatures. . .Our consciousness is meted out in chapters. . .Angels must wonder at these beings who fall so regularly out of awareness into a fantasm-infested dark. How our frail identities survive these chasms no philosopher has ever been able to explain.*
>
> (Iris Murdoch, *The Black Prince*, 1973: 231–2)

The French phenomenologist Merleau-Ponty is a common starting point, if not end point, when it comes to embodied themes and issues: a definitive source or reference point, in fact, providing a viable critique and alternative to Cartesian dualism in which mind and body are torn asunder.

Perception, Merleau-Ponty (1962) reminds us, is always from somewhere (never from nowhere), and that somewhere is grounded in our embodied being-in-the-world. I cannot, for example, when facing forward, see what is going on behind me, except with the aid of mirrors or technological trickery. Perception, therefore, is no God's eye phenomenon, it is entirely embodied in the here and now. Mind and body, indeed, contra Descartes, are inter-fused at the pre-objective, pre-reflective level of lived experience. Meaning, in turn, inheres in our embodied behaviours and gestures as part and parcel of our very being-in-the-world and the intentionality this entails. There is, moreover, a radical reversibility at work in all this. The seer, for example, can be seen, the hearer heard, the toucher touched and so on. Inter-subjectivity, in this respect, pertains to our dwelling in a common, shared or inter-mundane world, which itself involves a set of inter-corporeal relations. All this, however, presupposes the waking body-subject. Merleau-Ponty, in fact, has precious little to say on sleep or the sleeping body. There is enough here, nonetheless, for a phenomenological account of sleep to be recovered, fathomed or fashioned.

Leder (1990), for example, helps us do just that through his own phenomenological explorations of the *absent* body in general and the *ecstatic–recessive* body in particular. In the normal course of day-to-day events, Leder notes, the body projects *outwards* in experience, thereby steering attention away from its bodily points of origin: an *ecstatic* mode of being, that is to say, in which the body dis-appears, phenomenologically speaking, as an object of thematic experience. Existential events such as pain, of course, shatter any such state of affairs, the body instead *dys-appearing* as a problematic site of experience if not an alien 'it'. My ribs, for instance, suddenly hurt and hence dys-appear, when cracked or broken, in contrast to their normal modes of corporeal dis-appearance (Leder 1990). The very same point, perhaps, holds good with respect to tiredness, sleepiness and insomnia: further modes of bodily dys-appearance, that is to say.

Sleep, however, phenomenologically speaking, points us in the opposite (*recessive*) direction, involving what Leder terms 'depth disappearance'. That is to say, the body not only projects outwards (*ecstatically*) into the world, but 'falls back into *unexperiencable depths*' (1990: 53, my empha-sis). This depth, in turn, must be understood not simply in *spatial* terms but in *temporal* terms as a distinct (cyclical) phase of embodiment. Sleep, from this perspective, is a radical form of 'disappearance' or '*withdrawal* from experience' (1990: 57, original emphasis). Dreams, to be sure, as part or portion of sleep, may 'restore' an experiential process, but a 'preliminary severance' from waking involvements, Leder rightly notes, is necessary to dream. It is this 'severance', this *'loss of consciousness to the world* that is shared by all phases of sleep' (1990: 57).

A phenomenology of 'falling asleep', if not 'being asleep', provides further clues to the modes of (depth) disappearance involved here. Sleep, Merleau-Ponty notes, is not something I can directly will or intentionally call forth. I may 'look to sleep', 'mimic' sleep, ritually 'play' at sleep, or indirectly try to influence its occurrence in a variety of ingenious ways, but try as I might sleep comes of its own accord: a sort of 'descending' or 'coming over us', despite ourselves, the precise moment of which is difficult if not impossible to recall upon waking. Our very attempts to will sleep, moreover, may be self-defeating, resulting in unwelcome bouts of insomnia that leave us tired and weary[1]. Recounting his own attempts at sleep, for instance, Merleau-Ponty puts it like this:

> I lie down in bed, on my left side, with my knees drawn up: I close my eyes and breath slowly, putting my plans out of my mind. But the power of my will or consciousness stops there. As the faithful, in the Dionysian mysteries, invoke the god by miming scenes from his life, *I call up the visitation of sleep by imitating the breathing and posture of the sleeper.* The god is actually there when the faithful can no longer distinguish themselves from the part they are playing, when their body and their consciousness cease to bring in, as an obstacle, their particular opacity, and when they are totally fused in the myth. *There is a moment when sleep 'comes', settling on this imitation itself which I have been offering to it, and I succeed in becoming what I was trying to be.*
>
> (1962: 163–4, my emphases)[2]

Lying awake then, out of the active play of the world, puts my body in a state of 'background disappearance', yet sleep involves something far 'deeper' and far more mysterious. When I (finally) succumb to sleep a 'depth disappearance' enfolds my body in its entirety, including *loss of volitional control of my eyes, ears and limbs* (Leder 1990). No longer ectastic, in other words, the body is now recessed from my command, control and awareness. I no longer perceive my body, nor can I perceive from it:

> In deep sleep, interoception, proprioception, exteroception – all recede. My own sleeping body is something I will never directly see. Where 'it' is, 'I', as conscious, perceiving subject, necessarily, am not.
>
> (1990: 58)

We can only access the sleeping body, as this suggests, *indirectly*. Upon awakening, for example, I may fallibly piece together the nature, quality and quantity of my sleep (Leder 1990). How do I feel? Am I (still) tired? Did I get enough sleep? These are some of the questions I may ask myself when emerging from my slumber. Others too, of course, provide another indirect route into the nature and quality of our sleep life, whether our nearest and dearest or the technician in the sleep lab. As far as I am concerned, nonetheless, I cannot *directly* audit my own sleep. I am the one person, in fact, who will never (thankfully) 'hear myself snore', though my partner 'may describe it in no uncertain terms' (Leder 1990: 58) (of which more later). Sleep, therefore, involves a certain *'absence'* from both self and others, these *indirect* modes of recovery or apprehension notwithstanding. Most of the world, indeed, has never seen me sleep or, to put it another way, has only seen my waking or wakeful body-self (Leder 1990). The sleeping body thus partakes of all aspects of 'depth disappearance':

> It disappears from perception and command, from self and other, as a result of its withdrawal from the sensorimotor circuit. The complemental series constituted by body, surface and depth here exhibits a temporal dimension. I oscillate between the depth disappearance of sleep and the mixed modes characteristic of the waking self.
>
> (1990: 59)

Between 'deep sleep' and 'alert wakefulness', nonetheless, lie a range of 'intermediate positions' or 'transitional states' through which we 'cyclically move' (Leder 1990). These include 'light sleep', 'half sleep', dream states, and various other 'twilight' or 'hypnagogic' experiences (cf. Mavromatis 1987) – states, that is to say, somewhere between ecstasis (the 'I can') and recession (the 'I cannot') (Leder 1990: 57). People (recalling the discussion and definition of sleep in Chapter 1) are never entirely 'cut off' from or 'dead to the world' when asleep. Not only is sleep (rapidly) reversible, it also involves a highly *selective screening* or sensitivity to external stimuli. Some things may not wake us but others surely will: the gentle calling of our name, for instance, or the slightest stirrings or movements of a mother's newborn baby. A strong enough stimuli, if all else fails, will usually arouse us, and 'seize us back' into the waking world, happily or otherwise (Leder 1990). I may also, to complicate things further, go to bed at night, resolving to wake early the next morning with the aid of an alarm clock, only to find myself awakening unprompted at the appropriate time or thereabouts without the need for its ringing tones. In these and other ways, then, sleep is a *liminal*, betwixt and between state, hovering between consciousness and unconsciousness, the direct and the indirect, the voluntary and the involuntary. Our 'intentional threads to the intersubjective world', to paraphrase Merleau-Ponty, are 'never entirely severed', not even in the deepest, darkest moments of sleep.

In deep sleep nonetheless, Leder claims, we discover the 'radical anonymity of natural existence'. 'Nightly', I give myself over to those:

> . . .vegetative processes that form but a circumscribed region of my day-body. Surface functions will be all but abandoned, I become a creature of depth, lost in respiration, digestion, and circulation. My experiential world rests upon the restorative powers of this unconscious being. I can surface for only a limited time before requiring resubmergence in the impersonal.
>
> (1990: 59)

To call this a 'nightly' process, however, is to miss something important or significant. Sleep, of course, may take place day or night, or both, depending on a range of factors including age, employment and lifestyle. The 'day-body', in other words, is not necessarily synonymous with wakefulness any more than the 'night-body' is synonymous with sleep. Leder's general phenomenological contentions, nonetheless, hold good, at least as far as the sleeping or dormant body is concerned.

Further phenomenological echoes and insights into these dormant matters, particularly the *temporal* dimensions of sleep and dreams, can be gleaned through works such as Schutz's (1973) on *The Structures of the Lifeworld* (Schutz with Luckman 1974/1973).[3] In sleep, Schutz argues, through a 'radical alteration in the tension of consciousness, I withdraw from the intersubjective world'. Upon awakening, moreover, 'my activities of consciousness begin where they left off, before I went to sleep' (1973: 46). Prior to sleep, for instance:

> I made my mind up to jump out of bed early tomorrow immediately upon awakening. Now I confront this resolution (no matter what I have dreamt of in the interim). In this sense, I 'find' myself in the morning as I 'left' myself last evening. It at first appears that I am again connected with time of my waking life which was 'broken off' that evening. But between my withdrawal from the everyday life-world and my recent return to it, 'time has not stood still'. It has become morning. I experience the world as having become older (yesterday was Sunday, today is Monday). *I live through world time as transcending 'my' time*. This lived experience of transcendence, although an everyday one, concerns the world in general in its temporal structure.
>
> (1973: 46)

The 'transcendence of world time', in this respect, can be experienced in both the 'withdrawal into sleep' and the 'return to being awake': all this, moreover, 'without reference to the existence of fellow men [*sic*]' (1973: 46).

As for the time structure of the dream world, this Schutz reminds us, is 'extraordinarily complex': earlier, later, past, present and future all appear confounded, mixed or muddled (1973: 33). We can only 'grasp the sphere of dreams', moreover, by means of 'indirect communication', to use Kierkegaard's expression (Schutz 1973: 34). The poet or artist, in this respect, is:

> . . . far closer to a description adequate to the meaning of the dream world than the scientist and philosopher, since his [*sic*] means of communication attempt to transcend the everyday meaning, structure and language.
>
> (1973: 34)

No account of the phenomenology of sleep, particularly its spatial and temporal dimensions, would be complete without recourse to Proust, whose seminal seven-volume work – *A la recherché du temp perdu* (*In search of lost time* or *Remembrance of things past*) – is literally packed with references to these dormant matters (2002). Proust loved sleep, by all accounts, and was passionate about his bed (see Chapter 2). The opening pages of Vol I: *Swan's Way*, for instance, plunge us deep into these phenomenological waters. 'For a long time', the narrator tells us: 'I would go to bed early. Sometimes, the candle barely out, my eyes closed so quickly that I did not have time to tell myself: "I'm falling asleep". And half an hour later the thought that it was *time to look for sleep* would awaken me' (2002: 1). When a man is asleep, the narrator continues, 'he has around him the chain of the hours, the sequence of the years, the order of the heavenly bodies. Instinctively he consults them when he awakes, and in an instant reads off his own position on the earth's surface and the time that has elapsed during his slumbers; but this ordered procession is apt to grow confused, and to break its ranks' (2002: 3–4). For Proust's narrator, nonetheless, in all probability himself, it was 'enough' if:

> . . . in my own bed, my sleep was so heavy as completely to relax my consciousness; for then I lost all sense of the place in which I had gone to sleep, and when I awoke in the middle of the night, not knowing where I was, I could not *even be sure at first who I was*; I had *only the most rudimentary sense of existence*, such as may lurk and flicker in the depths of an animals consciousness; *I was more destitute than a cave-dweller*, but then the memory. . . would come like a rope let down from heaven to draw me up out of the *abyss of not-being*, from which I could never have escaped by myself.
>
> (2002: 4)

Magical stuff indeed! These and many other sleep-related insights pulse through Proust's meditations on time and memory, love and loss, art and artistic vocation. A phenomenology of sleep, in short, Proustian or otherwise, helps us recover or reclaim, if not reconceptualize, our cyclical (ad)ventures into this great 'abyss of oblivion' or 'not-being'. 'To be or not to be?': that indeed is the question.

The '(un)doing' of slee*ping*: Parsons, Goffman and beyond. . .

Where then do we go from here? How can we take these phenomenological insights forward into a more fully-fledged or fleshed-out sociological account?

A useful starting point is to see sleep itself, in sociological terms, as a crucial form or mechanism of 'social release'; what Schwartz (1970) appositely terms a 'periodic remission' from the conscious demands of waking society or, to put it slightly differently, a case of sleep as 'sanctuary' or 'salvation'. Without such 'periodic remission', Schwartz declares, social life would quite simply be intolerable if not impossible. If sleep disappeared overnight, we would surely be obliged to find some 'functional equivalent' for it, sociologically speaking (1970: 486). This, of course, is no major new sociological insight. Samuel Johnson, for example, noted something similar way back in the eighteenth century:

> Let him that desires most have all his desires gratified, he never shall attain a state, which he can, for a day and a night, contemplate with satisfaction, or from which, *if he had the power of perpetual vigilance, he would not long for periodical separations.*
>
> (Johnson 2003/1739–61: *The Idler*, No. 32
> Saturday, 25 November 1758, my emphasis)

It does nonetheless provide us with an important sociological lead or point of departure as far as sleep is concerned. Parsons, for instance, in a tantalisingly brief sociological comment, puts it like this:

> It is inherent in the view of social action taken here that all such action involves tensions and the necessity of the imposition of frustrations and disciplines of the most various sorts. This fact underlies the occurrence of a variety of rhythmic cycles of effort and rest, of discipline and permissive release and the like. *Sleep is clearly one of the most fundamental of these tension release phenomena, which though it has biological foundations is nevertheless profoundly influenced by interaction on the socio-cultural levels.*
>
> (1951: 396, my emphasis)

Sleep, for this very reason, is a socially scheduled, socially organised and socially institutionalised pursuit or practice. This in turn raises the intriguing sociological possibility of something akin to the *'sleep role'* involving a reciprocal cluster of *rights* and *responsibilities* on the part of the sleeper, as occupant or incumbent of the sleep role, and other waking members of society alike, particularly those with whom the sleeper is sufficiently co-present for mutual interference to occur (Schwartz 1970). The sleep role, to be sure, is socially, culturally and historically variable. Viewed through the lens of contemporary (monophasic – see Chapter 4) Western society, however, it is *likely* to include the following:

Rights:

- Exemption from normal role obligations/relinquishing of conscious waking involvement in society[4].
- Freedom from interruption from other (waking) members of society, except in times of emergency.
- No loss of waking role status whilst asleep.

Responsibilities:

- To conform to the general pattern of sleep time, unless legitimate social circumstances, such as work arrangements, dictate otherwise.
- To sleep in a bed, or similar device, in a private place, away from public view (a maximum of two per bed is the general norm).

Whether or not sleep is 'the' fundamental tension release phenomenon that Schwartz implies – a 'total' release and the most 'radical' form of periodic withdrawal, in his view, from the social world 'outside us' and the society 'within us' (cf. Cooley 1902) – is a moot point. The perceptual wall that sleep erects between us and the outside world, as already noted, is *selective* rather than absolute and we are never entirely 'cut off' from the inter-subjective world, however soundly we sleep. Dreams, moreover, may or may not violate the 'totality' of sleep's 'conscious remission'. Certainly, as Schwartz suggests, dreams are remissive if not transgressive with respect to 'normative constraints', but different types of (lucid) dreams, let alone different types of (light–deep) sleep, add a further layer of complexity to these debates.

The sleep role, nonetheless, is far from unproblematic, or perhaps more correctly uncontested, cast in Parsonian terms at least. Compared to other social roles, it is certainly a-typical, not least because its incumbent remains (blissfully) unaware of this role occupancy *qua* sleeper when asleep. Whilst certain useful analogies, moreover, may be drawn between the Parsonian sick role and the Parsonian sleep role – the fact that sleep, like illness, for instance, is simultaneously a bodily state and a social status, the fact that sleep is a therapy of sorts, and the fact that power differentials between sleeping and waking agents replicate, in part at least, those between doctors and patients (Crossley 2004) – caution is needed with respect to the sleep role ideal, given that these very rights and responsibilities are claimed but contested in social life. These rights and responsibilities must, in other words, as Crossley astutely observes, 'be won' and, in some cases, 'renegotiated' in what will inevitably be a local, contingent, interactional context of 'power and conflict': more a question of (strategic) interaction and on-going negotiation, that is to say, than any fixed role prescriptions (2004: 20). Add to this the potential 'unravelling' of any such rights and responsibilities in the so-called 24/7 era, and the picture becomes far more complicated than may first appear[5].

The sleep role then, is a useful sociological concept *both* to think *with* and *against*. It also raises a series of further intriguing sociological possibilities. Adopting the sleep role, for example, *qua* social act or status, is far from synonymous with sleep in the biological or psycho-physiological sense of the word (Schwartz 1970). I may, for instance, to all intents and purposes, be treated, and expect to be treated, as socially 'asleep' even when I am biologically awake. I may also, of course, feign sleep in order to hood-wink somebody or to excuse or absolve myself from some taxing, tricky, troubling or just plain boring social situation.

The meaning and legitimacy of sleep, in turn, is *socially variable* and *contextually dependent*. In legitimate circumstances, for instance, the sleeper's sleep is usually honoured or respected. In other 'illegitimate' circumstances, such as you or I falling asleep at an important event or occasion, it may be greeted with disapproval or stern rebuke. The notion of '(in)appropriate' sleep, if not 'anarchic', 'anomic', 'deviant' or 'stigmatised' sleep roles (Schwartz 1970), also springs to mind here, which covers a multitude of sins, from falling asleep at the wheel, through the unpredictable sleep attacks of narcoleptics, the sleeping patterns of night-shift workers, to the 'rough' sleeper on the streets. Here we encounter a further important sociological insight, already touched on in Chapter 2, namely that *when* we sleep, *where* we sleep and *with whom* we sleep are all important markers or indicators of social status, privilege and prevailing power relations – an issue we shall elaborate upon more fully in the next chapter.

A turn from Parsonian to Goffmanesque themes is instructive at this point, adding further important sociological insights on sleep within the 'interaction order'. Goffman, like most other sociologists, has precious little to say directly on these matters. His sparkling sociological concepts and insights, nonetheless, lend themselves nicely to various aspects of sleep, as Schwartz (1970) rightly notes, in particular the 'doing' of slee*ping* in everyday/everynight life – the *meanings*, *methods*, *motives* and *management* of sleep, that is to say (Taylor 1993). Sleeping, from this perspective, may be construed as a *main* or *side*, *dominant* or *subordinate* involvement (Goffman 1963; Steger and Brunt 2003), depending on the circumstances in question. To the extent that the individual physically withdraws to a quiet place with the sole purpose of sleeping, for instance, we may speak of sleeping as a *main* or *dominant* involvement – an *all-engrossing* event or prime concern. Sleep, however, may take the form of a *side involvement*, such as napping on the train: the main or dominant purpose being the train journey and getting off at the right stop (Steger 2003a; Steger and Brunt 2003: 19)!

As for the notion of sleeping as a *subordinate involvement*, one need look no further than the Japanese art of *inemuri*. The main characteristic or defining feature of *inemuri*, Steger and Brunt explain, is that 'the sleeper is present in a situation which is *meant for something other than sleep*' (2003: 1, my emphasis). It is quite customary and acceptable it seems, in Japanese society at least, to doze or drop off at a lecture, a meeting, a party or other social occasion or gathering without incurring any social sanction or disapproval. *Inemuri*, however, socially speaking, cannot be regarded as being completely 'out of play' or 'dead to the world'. The individual indeed must be ready to relinquish his or her 'sleep' at the appropriate moment (hence the notion of a *subordinate* involvement) when the dominant involvement demands or dictates active participation. *Inemuri*, then, may be construed as a 'light' or 'quasi-sleep state' and a *subordinate involvement* to the main event or occasion, whether a party or some other such gathering or event. *Inemuri*, moreover, as we shall see in the next chapter, is itself a 'special case' of a broader phenomenon in Japanese society, one which has proved resistant to Western 'ideals' of the eight-hour *monophasic* sleep pattern; namely, a *polyphasic* sleep or *napping* culture (Steger 2003a; Steger and Brunt 2003). We may indeed go one or more steps further here and propose the seemingly counter-intuitive notion of the *'socially attentive sleeper'*, particularly in cases where sleep remains a subordinate involvement[6]. Relations between the socially attentive and the *socially (in)considerate sleeper*, in turn, add a further layer of complexity to these debates, of which more later.

Matters do not end here, however. The partaking of sleep, or perhaps more correctly the partaking of socially legitimate sleep, usually requires something akin to a 'transition phase' whereby the individual gradually moves into and out of this role (Schwartz 1970). The sleeper, in other words, continuing these Goffmanesque themes, is protected by an 'interactional membrane' (cf. Goffman 1961a) which reliably 'filters out disturbing communications' at points of *entry* and *exit* from the sleep role (Schwartz 1970: 489). This in turn allows people to properly 'wind down' from or 'warm up' to the demands of waking life, including what may be an elaborate series of bedtime routines, rites or rituals such as brushing one's teeth, undressing, warm baths, milky drinks, putting on one's night-time attire, reading, listening to the radio, meditation or prayers, and waking routines such as showering, shaving, dressing, having breakfast and so forth.

What we have here then is a *status* or *role passage*, which itself is mediated or facilitated by a 'transition phase' or 'interactional membrane' of the utmost importance for any successful or accomplished, dignified if not distinguished, movement to and from the waking world. Pre- and post-sleep routines, rituals or habits, in this respect – themselves yet another (reflexive) dimension of body-techniques and habitus (cf. Bourdieu 1984, 1990, 2000; Crossley 2001, 2004; Mauss 1973/1934) – are part and parcel of the *active* 'doing' and 'undoing' of sleeping, which itself, to repeat, includes the *methods, motives* and *management* of sleeping in everyday/everynight life, as well as the *meanings* we attribute to it (Taylor 1993). Sleep, from this perspective, is itself mediated by way of (reflexive) body techniques which bring it under our own partial control (Crossley 2004): a powerful reminder once again of the purposive as well as the non-purposive, personal as well as pre-personal elements of this embodied transition both into and out of existence as conscious waking beings. It is not simply a question of the individual preparing for bed because they are tired or sleepy, moreover, but of *growing tired* or *sleepy* in and through these preparatory phases, processes or practices themselves: a 'reciprocity of motive and action in the sleep role', as Schwartz appositely puts it (1970: 488–91). These techniques and rituals in turn provide a crucial means of establishing ontological security and basic trust (cf. Giddens 1991), which themselves are important prerequisites or ingredients for the effectiveness of those very techniques and rituals (Crossley 2004: 11). Again we glimpse something of the learnt/ habitual/reflexive dimensions of sleep, or perhaps more correctly our passage into and out of it: a topic we shall return to shortly.

So far so good, but to really bring these insights 'to life', so to speak, we need to see how they are put into practice or played out across the life course: a process in which biographical themes and embodied issues to do with 'growing up' and 'growing old' loom large.

Sleep across the life course: from childhood to (deep) old age. . .

We may well have 'time-transcending' minds – if by that we mean the ability to think beyond the temporal horizons of our own fleshy mortal casing – but we still nonetheless have 'time-bound bodies' which age, decline and die (Bauman 1992). Sleep too is known to vary in more or less predictable ways throughout our lifetimes, from conception or cradle, through childhood, youth and (early) adulthood to (deep) old age. Sleep science, for example, tells us that the (dreaming) foetus spends most of its time immersed in precursor REM (or active) sleep, hence the kicking and twitching in the mother's womb. Several years later, however, the self-same individual will have a very different architecture of sleep. REM sleep will constitute a much smaller proportion of total sleep time, and much less time will be spent asleep (Martin 2003: 221). In fact, more of our sleep time as we age is made up of the shallower stages of 1 and 2 of NREM. Slow-wave sleep, in other words, declines with age from about 20–25 per cent of total sleep in early childhood to less than five per cent by middle age, with older people getting precious little slow-wave sleep (Bliwise 2000: 26; Morgan 1987: Ch. 2). Sleep too becomes more fragmented with advancing years, with more frequent awakenings and a circadian shift to a more 'lark-like' pattern (Martin 2003: 237). In short, the 14–16-hours-a-day sleep average of young babies (of which about half is precursor REM or active sleep), or the 12–14-hours-a-day sleep average of the six month old infant (whose presursor REM or active sleep has now dropped to the adult level of approximately 25 per cent), is a far cry, quite literally, from the architecture of sleep in old age. Men, moreover, physiologically speaking, seem to show greater deterioration in their sleep architecture with age than women, including a higher percentage of lighter sleep stages (Morgan 1987; Reidiech et al 1990); an intriguing finding given the gendered nature of sleep disruption (of which more below). All this without any mention of complicating factors such as health status, or the 'owl-like' patterns of 'yawning youth'.

Again, this is merely a starting point. The underlying physiological mechanisms or hidden architecture of sleep, to be sure, may well vary in these more or less predictable ways over an individual's lifetime, but there is more, as we have already seen, to people's sleep than this, young or old, infant or infirm, male or female. Individuals differ considerably in their characteristic sleep patterns, and some of us need (far) more sleep than others. Research, Martin (2003: 222) comments, has 'barely begun to scratch the surface' of understanding *how* the manifold constituents of nature and nurture, biology and society, mind and body, combine to shape our individual sleep characteristics, and 'why yours are different from mine'[7]. That sleep is a complex, emergent, irreducible product of these factors, nonetheless, is surely beyond doubt. An *embodied* perspective on sleep across the life course, therefore, which incorporates, yet goes beyond, these biological or physiological considerations has much to contribute here. Placing sleep (disruption) in the context of people's (normal) day-to-day or night-to-night lives, including changing social roles, responsibilities and relationships across the life course augments previous phenomenological themes and sociological insights. This, in turn, brings into play relevant bodies of literature such as the sociology of childhood and the sociology of ageing, from which further insights concerning the '(un)doing' or negotiation of sleeping can be gleaned or garnered.

Children and childhood: the golden years of sleep?

The sociology of childhood has done much, in recent years, to reconceptualise our approaches to, and understandings of, children and childhoods, including attempts to *recontextualise* children *within* and *beyond* their families[8]. Not only must childhood or childhood*s* be understood as socially, culturally and historically variable, but children themselves must be seen as *active constructors* and *negotiators* of their own embodied lives, identities and relationships, with adults and with other children, across the public–private divide, albeit with varying degrees of success given structural facilitators and constraints[9]. The notion of children as a 'minority social group' in an adult-centric world is thrown into critical relief here, itself refracted and reflected through the intersections of *generation* and *gender*, thereby bringing children's rights to the fore (Mayall 1996, 2002). 'Work' too needs rethinking in this light. Children and young people play a vital role in the division of labour, including paid and unpaid, formal and informal work in the public and private spheres (Mayall 1996, 2002; Mizen et al 1999, 2001; Stacey 1988).

The '(un)doing' or negotiation of sleeping in children's lives, I venture, lends further support to these contentions, adding important new directions to the sociology of childhood in so doing. Sleep in fact provides a valuable new window onto the embodied lives of children, telling us much about their (inter)generational relations and their status or positioning within the social order and across the public–private divide (cf. also Elias' 1978/1939 insights into these issues in Chapter 2 in this book). It is also, of course, a significant barometer of social change as far as children and young people's own use of *time*, at home and at school is concerned.

A number of comments and observations may be made here in advancing these propositions. First, sleep is an important part of children's lives, like it or not; not simply in terms of health, growth, development and well-being (children quite literally 'grow up' in their sleep through the release of growth hormones), but in terms of the sheer amount of time devoted to it, in the early years at least. By early school age, for example, the average child will have spent 'more time sleeping than engaging in any other activity, including playing, social interaction and exploring the environment' (Wiggs 2004: 2).

Second, sleep involves important *learnt* components from early infancy onwards. Children's sleep, in this respect, not only provides us with a rich and fascinating opportunity to study its social *pliability* or *plasticity* – incorporated through the dormant habitus and associated body-techniques (cf. Bourdieu 1984, 1990, 2000; Elias 1978/1939; Mauss 1973/1934) – but also to understand sleep in *dynamic*, *relational* terms, including the reciprocal influence of family members upon each other's sleep. It is not simply, in other words, a case of parental influences upon children's sleep, good or bad, but of children's influence on other family members' sleep, including parents and siblings.

The third point returns us to the notion of children's 'minority group' status. Sleep is a key site in which inter-generational power relations and issues of authority, autonomy and independence are played out. Children, for example, by and large, have far less *decision-making latitude* over sleep than adults. The nature and quality of their sleep, moreover, is more or less keenly *watched over* or *worried about*, *monitored* or *managed*, by parents and professionals alike, including the most intimate, frightening or embarrassing of incidents such as bed-wetting, night terrors and nocturnal emissions: a level of watchfulness that adults themselves, if positions were reversed, would doubtless find uncomfortable if not downright irritating or invasive in all but the most exceptional circumstances. This, however, has its *pros* as well as it *cons*. Whilst many children and young people, indeed, find parental (most likely maternal) worry about these and other matters, inside and outside the home, irritating and constraining, they also see it as 'part and parcel of being proper parents, symbolizing concern' (Brannen and O'Brien 1996: 7; cf. Allatt 1996).

A fourth point pertains to the intersections of time and space in *siting* or *situating* children's sleep. It is not simply, as this suggests, a question of *when* and *how* children sleep, or *who* is doing the watching or worrying, but of *where* they sleep. The location or siting of children's sleep reveals yet another important dimension of children's situation and social status. Where and when children sleep, for example, both *inside* and *outside* the home, is a key issue in family life and child–adult relations, from co-sleeping practices, accommodation arrangements and bedroom space at home, to the negotiation of overnight stays, sleep-over parties and the like with friends. Within the family home, for instance, a sibling pecking order of sleeping places and spaces may well be apparent, with older children having their own rooms, and younger children making-do with a shared bedroom, if not bunk beds. This in turn, of course, relates to the material circumstances and socio-economic status of the family. Mayall (2002), for example, recounts a revealing exchange with Gamse – a nine-year-old girl who lives with her parents and four siblings in a two-bedroom council flat. Both parents, Mayall tells us, are busy with childcare and running a shop. Asking whether Gamse shares a room, she replies:

> Yes I do. Because I live in a small council flat. My brother has his own room, it's very small and you can't even fit in. My Mum and Dad sleep on the sofa bed in the sitting room, and me and my sister sleep in bunk beds and the twins in their cots in my bedroom as well. . ... It works out fine. I would prefer the sofa bed. Sometimes when my Dad comes home late, I get in there, and then when he comes in I get in my own bed.
>
> (quoted in Mayall 2002: 42–3)

When families do not all live 'under the same roof', moreover, then children's sleeping places and spaces may rapidly multiply, including stays with separated parents (usually dads) and/or with grandparents. This, for example, was a common theme in our own pilot work on children and sleep

(Williams, Griffiths and Lowe 2004). So too were stay-overs at friends' houses, particularly at weekends. A thirteen-year-old girl, for example, made the following entry in her sleep diary:

> Saturday 10:20am: Last night I slept at Nina's house, my best friend who lives two doors away. We were laughing and joking until 12:30, then we got into bed, and I slept from that point until 6:45 when I woke up sneezing (hayfever). I fell asleep again but woke up 3 times, 7:10, 7:45, 8:30 before I finally got up with Nina at about 9:30 when the alarm went off.

As for children's own responsibilities for the sleeping or waking of others, Gamse's comments are again instructive:

> . . .in the morning, I'm responsible for waking my sister up. My brother wakes himself up, 'cos 8 o'clock he goes to school, and in the morning my Mum sleeps in. So it's my responsibility to wake up and wake Mary up and get her breakfast and get her ready. . .
> (quoted in Mayall 2002: 44)

Gamse's life, in this respect, including, to repeat her, *sleeping life*, is 'structured through the family's housing and the busy working lives of both parents, mediated by her parents' decisions on how childhood should be lived in the local context' (Mayall 2002: 44).

As children grow up, and their roles and responsibilities change, bargaining, negotiation or outright unilateral decision making about sleep time is likely to increase. Discretion or decision-making latitude over sleep-time, in this respect, echoing an earlier point, is itself a prime marker of social status if not a rite of passage. Indeed, sleep may well be seen as a 'boring' or 'uncool' topic in the eyes of many children today, and being 'sent to bed' or told to 'be in by' a certain time a social sanction they could well do without, but concerns are growing amongst sleep experts and other interested parties that children are not getting enough sleep. Excessive (subjective) daytime sleepiness, for example, according to various studies, is a common problem amongst children of school age, students and young adults (see Wiggs 2004 for a general review of the evidence and Chapter 4 in this book).

One line of thinking here is that the 'pre-sleep' activities of modern-day children have changed. Televisions, computers and other forms of entertainment, for example, are commonly found in children's bedrooms (Owens et al 1999; Van den Bulck 2004)[10]. As these new 'childhood' pre-sleep activities become more widespread, so the more traditional (calming, relaxing) ones such as reading or being read to, have declined (Wiggs 2004: 3). They are also, of course, relatively 'unstructured' activities without clearly defined start and end points; activities furthermore which are not 'compensated' for at other points in the week(end) (Van den Bulck 2004). The current vogue or penchant for text-messaging at any time of the day or night adds another important dimension to the picture of 'yawning youth' (Van den Bulck 2003). Children, so the argument goes, are 'increasingly being bombarded with electronic stimulation until lights go out'. ' "Go to bed" ', moreover, 'may no longer mean "go to sleep", but rather "go to your bedroom and amuse yourself until you get so tired that you fall asleep with the video still running"' (Wiggs 2004: 4). These digital or electronic pressures, it is argued, in association with broader transformations and contradictions in youth culture today, make for a complex picture of cross-cutting influences, which, taken together, give cause for concern.

References to things such as television were certainly common in our own pilot work on children and sleep (Williams, Griffiths and Lowe 2004). So too were other sources of distraction, disturbance or disruption such as noisy, boisterous or needy siblings. A thirteen-year-old girl, for example, made the following sleep diary entry:

> Tuesday 7:15am: Last night I decided *not* to watch the late Big Brother (Channel 4 TV show) so I went to bed at 10:00pm. I started to sleep but Connor [brother] kept on running in and making me jump and wake up (he was filling me in on what was happening on TV). After four times he stopped and I finally got to sleep at 10:20pm. I woke up when my alarm went off at 6:45am, but I fell back to sleep until 7:00am. Apart from that I was not disturbed.

Another fifteen year-old girl writes:

> Monday night: I went to my room at 11:10pm after Big Brother. By the time I got into bed and began to nod off it was 11:25 but then my little sister came in and said she couldn't sleep, so *I got up and put her back to bed*. I finally fell asleep at about 11:40 and got up when my alarm went off at 7:10am.

Again we glimpse here the complexities of children's sleep lives, including the influence of sibling relations and responsibilities within the home. It is important in fully accounting for children's sleep time, to also examine broader trends in the division of labour and the 'redistribution of responsibilities'. Children, Mayall (2002: 64) comments, find themselves ever more 'scholarised' (as learners not workers) with 'free time reduced both in and out of school'. The paid work of children, moreover, from newspaper rounds in the early morning to Saturday jobs, puts further pressure on children's sleep time, to say nothing of other unpaid work and family responsibilities of the kind mentioned above (Mizen et al 1999). American children, in this respect, may well be experiencing later school start-times for that extra hour in bed on school days (Epstein 1998)[11], but there is a long way to go, so we are told, in order to relieve if not reverse these trends in children's sleep patterns and practices. These are issues we shall return to in the next two chapters, including the 'problem' of tired or sleepy children and childhood sleep 'disorders' from sleep apnoea to night-terrors and soggy sheets. Suffice to say, in the present context, that children's sleep is increasingly problematised if not pathologised, with links not simply to health, happiness and well-being, but to their behaviour, intelligence and academic performance. The golden years of sleep, from this viewpoint, may not be quite so golden after all.

Listening to children's voices nonetheless remains an important yet neglected aspect of these (adult-centric, top-down) debates to date; another dimension of their marginal or minority group status. We should also, of course, at one and the same time, recognise the importance not simply of inter-generational relations but of variations amongst children themselves according to factors such as class, gender and ethnicity. Children, it is clear, are a far from homogenous group. Boys, for example, may *view* if not *do* sleep quite differently to girls. This in turn may vary according to different types of masculinity, class and ethnic background. Strategies for managing sleep(iness) are also likely to vary according to factors such as age. Teenagers, for instance, who tend to go to bed later as they get older, may 'compensate' by sleeping in late at weekends and during vacations, and/or get through on caffeine-laced (soft) drinks (Martin 2003). It is tempting indeed, rightly or wrongly, to characterize youth culture as one in which lack of sleep is the 'norm', something to be bragged or boasted about even, with too much sleep denounced as 'boring', 'dull', 'deviant' or 'nerd-like'.

A peek into the changing night-scene of Japanese youth culture sheds further light (no pun intended) on these issues. Nowadays, Ayukawa (2003) tells us, young people in Japan stay up much later than previously. When at home, they engage in activities such as listening to music, accessing the Internet, talking to/texting friends with their mobile phones, or watching TV. In September 2001 an enterprising English school took advantage of this trend through the provision of late-night English lessons online from 10.30pm to 7.30am (2003: 149). Outside the home, moreover, young people 'walk around the streets or congregate at convenience stores and karioke boxes, and young women especially also engage in telephone dating services which sometimes lead them to disappear from home for a period of time' (2003: 149). Relationships in this respect, Ayukawa argues, have become more 'fluid' and 'temporary' and boundaries between conventional and deviant behaviours have become blurred if not redrawn: passports to a 'new world', in effect, which allow for 'new behaviour, new ways of thinking and new perspectives on youth and youth cultures' (2003: 149).

Pressures to squeeze or skip sleep, of course, become even greater once young people leave the family home to go to college or university, or to start work. Most studies, in fact, attest to this pattern, which, if the statistics are anything to go by, appears to be getting worse. The average daily sleep duration of college students, for example, is estimated to have dropped by one hour in the past twenty years (Martin 2003: 236). To 'party on', in this respect, in association with the pressures of work or study, has its downside as well as its upside as far as sleep is concerned, not least when the effects of alcohol and recreational drug use are weighed in the balance (see also Chapter 4).

(Early) adulthood to mid-life: disruption and decline?

Early adulthood may be a time when people are 'footloose and fancy free', relatively speaking: a time perhaps, compared to later years, when one burns the candle at both ends, successfully or otherwise. Early patterns of family formation add another dimension to the picture, as all weary parents know!

Brannen and Moss's (1988) study of new mothers at work, for example, is revealing on this count. Tiredness, they note, is a major feature of these women's experience, which varies in quality as well as quantity according to different stresses in different circumstances and situations. Young babies and disturbed nights, for example, led to one type of tiredness; being at home all day was likely to bring a different type of tiredness associated with lethargy and boredom (a product of repetitive domestic chores and routines unbroken by much social contact); trying to combine domestic and paid work resulted in another type of tiredness through physical and mental fatigue. Certain forms of tiredness, moreover, were preferred to others. Some women, for instance, preferred feeling physically tired from working hard to feeling lethargic at home. As one woman put it:

> I used to feel tired because I was indoors. You can go to bed and sleep. It's through actually *doing* something rather than being stuck in the house. I'm usually tired in the evening by the time I get home and sort everything out. I don't usually sit down very early, but by the time I do I feel quite worn out.
>
> (Clerk, aged 22, quoted in Brannen and Moss 1988: 120)

Popay (1990) provides further insights into these issues in her own study of tiredness, including the accounts of both women and men in the case-study households. Most respondents commented on tiredness at some point during the interviews, but the women were more likely to do so than men (see also Hochschild with Machung 1990)[12]. More importantly, however, two different types of tiredness emerged, themselves gendered. The first type, evident in all but two of the men's accounts and five of the women's accounts, presented tiredness as a 'minor or intermittent event which was a normal part of life and basically not a cause for concern' (Popay 1990: 107). Amongst men, in particular, this was linked to paid work, either in terms of the *hours* or the *pressures* of work:

> Over the last 4–5 years the *hours have got longer.* . .I don't particularly mind the week. . .. I do find at weekends I sleep quite a lot. . .. It's quite tiring, especially if you go out in the evening. I mean you find yourself awake from 6.30 'til. . .I mean I've got to bed last night at one o'clock. . .. Some people can do it, I can't. So I get quite tired.
>
> (father, quoted in Popay 1990: 107)

The second type of tiredness, in contrast, was commented on by most women and two men. Here, tiredness was described as a *severe* or *chronic* experience. These accounts were provided by women with very different household situations in terms of the number and age of children, their employment status and their standard of living:

> The worst thing is tiredness, the exhaustion. . .by the end of the day. . .you're too physically exhausted to do anything.
>
> (part-time employed mother in a high-income household of two parents and three children aged 6 months, 3 years, 6 years, quoted in Popay 1990: 108)

Although women with older children did report severe tiredness, some of the most 'vivid and extreme accounts' of physical and mental exhaustion, echoing Brannen and Moss's (1988) findings, were provided by women with young children either talking about their current experiences or in relation to the period when their children were small. Two prominent themes here, in addition to 'broken nights', appeared to be the 'constant demands made on one's time and energy by small children and the responsibility one has for their welfare and development' (Popay 1990: 110). As one woman put it:

> Thomas couldn't go to bed unless he was breast fed and I was exhausted and didn't feel like doing it and it just seemed like all on me. . .he was big enough really to go to bed on his own, but it was just like a *habit* and. . .he was still acting like a baby. . .. You're *always alert.* . .not completely relaxed. . .*even when they're sleeping.* . .because you feel it is your *responsibility.*
>
> (mother quoted in Popay 1990: 110)

This last reference to always being alert and having feelings of (around-the-clock) responsibility provide telling testimony, not simply to the disruption but the 'retuning' of women's sleep following childbirth and the transition to motherhood: one in which the (slightest) stirring of the sleeping infant or child is enough to awaken the mother *qua* socially attentive or socially attuned sleeper. In only a few instances, Popay reports, had severe tiredness triggered a visit to the doctor however. For this to occur, it seems tiredness had to be combined with other symptoms (1990: 108; see also Chapter 5 in this book).

As 'mid-life'(a fuzzy, fluid or contested term admittedly) approaches, a further series of life course tensions or transitions impact on the nature and quality of our sleep time, again in gendered ways. Mid-life women, Hislop and Arber argue, provide a 'critical test case for the study of the influence of gender roles and relationships on sleep' (2003a: 696). As well as experiencing the physiological symptoms of the menopause, for example, mid-life women may be re-entering the workforce on a full- or part-time basis after parenting, and rising to responsible positions with increasing stresses and pressures. They may also be supporting partners through periods of workplace change, redundancy, retirement, or experiencing relationship breakdown. As daughters of ageing parents, moreover, they may have 'increased caring responsibilities and the stresses of bereavement' (2003a: 696). Whilst each of these factors can result in sleep disturbance, it is the 'merging of these roles in mid-life', Hislop and Arber claim, which may 'increase the potential for deterioration in women's sleep'. The gendered nature of these roles and responsibilities, in turn, may contribute 'significantly to sleep disruption, with women fulfilling their commitment to the well-being of their families often to the detriment of their own sleep needs and rights' (2003a: 697).

It is not so much a question of the *quantity* or *duration* of women's sleep, however, Hislop and Arber show, but of its *quality*. This appears to be what matters most. A 'good' night's sleep, from this perspective, is characterized by a night 'free of disturbances, and a feeling of refreshment on waking'. For most women in the study, nonetheless, a good night's sleep in these terms was rare. As one respondent put it:

> I have things going round and round in my head and I can't go to sleep. I just feel so much better if I actually get a good night's sleep.
>
> (quoted in Hislop and Arber 2003a: 699)

The reality of mid-life women's sleep then, according to Hislop and Arber, is 'predominantly one of disruption, which may relate to difficulty falling asleep, intermittent waking during the night, lying awake unable to go back to sleep, and/or waking early' (2003a: 699). The search for a good night's sleep, furthermore, may actually involve women 'giving up their right to sleep in their own private sleeping place' (2003a: 699). This disruption may be a product of the 'physical and emotional labour involved in caring for children and young babies, as well as by teenage children coming in late, menopausal symptoms, waking up to go to the toilet, partner's snoring or restlessness, work or environmental factors' (2003a: 701). The physical and emotional labour involved in caring for other members of the family's sleep needs or problems, for instance, is well illustrated by the case of one women whose 10-year-old daughter suffered from frequent bed-wetting episodes. This, Hislop and Arber (2003a: 703) recount, involved the following tasks, duties and responsibilities: alertness during the night, responding to her daughter's calls for help, comforting her daughter, changing her daughter's clothing and bed linen, reassuring her child and getting her back to sleep, worrying about the psychological and/or physical reasons for her child's bed-wetting[13].

When problems overlap, moreover, the likelihood of sleep disturbance increases:

> I have no normal sleep pattern, it has gone. I have a baby that sleeps two hours less than any other baby, and then I get woken up by my (teenage) daughter who comes stumbling in drunk in the middle of the night, knocking things over and turning her music on too loud.
>
> (quoted in Hislop and Arber 2003a: 700)

Problems, indeed, can quickly mount or multiply, in a spiralling 'downward' fashion:

> Problems just seem enormous. Our mothers (my husband's and mine) have been recently widowed and are now on the state pension, either end of the country. We haven't got a car, and they are quite demanding. My son. . .is a disaster. (I've got) a job that is becoming more and more stressful. There seems less and less time for me.
>
> (quoted in Hislop and Arber 2003a: 700)

Women, however, were not simply passive in the face of these problems. A range of *strategies* to improve women's sleep quality and maximize sleep resources were evident amongst Hislop and Arber's respondents, including early evening exercise, spending quiet time alone, listening to music, writing a journal, reading, having a hot drink, relaxing through deep breathing, listening to comedy tapes, or (temporarily or permanently) relocating to another room when partner-induced sleep disturbance proved 'too much' or 'intolerable' (2003a: 705).

Sleep disturbance, then, as this suggests, is an inextricable part of these mid-life women's social realities. The quality of their sleep, as such, is 'structured by a multiplicity of roles and responsibilities they carry out as part of their daily lives; as partners and/or mothers, as working women, and as daughters of ageing parents' (Hislop and Arber 2003a: 709). Women, these authors conclude, are 'disadvantaged' as far as the 'right' to sleep goes. In short, being female within a family structure is associated with a 'loss of sleep rights' (2003a: 709).

This may well be so, but some further comments and observations on men, masculinities and sleep are nonetheless called for at this juncture. How do different types of work impact on men's sleep across the life course? How do men 'do' sleep? What role do different masculinities play here? These and many other questions remain to be answered, in sociological terms at least, given the limited work to date. Clues can be found however in the extant literature on men and masculinities through a close re-reading with sleep in mind. Watson's (2000) study of 'male bodies', for example, is suggestive on this count. Masculinity, he notes, is embodied in a variety of ways within an individual and his social environment, including *normative* (ideal), *pragmatic* (practical), *experiential* (feeling) and *visceral* (physical) dimensions or modes of embodiment. For most of Watson's participants, however, the key level of embodiment and the primary mode of agency in the social world was *pragmatic*: a functional mode of construction according to the socially ordered and ordering male gender roles of 'father', 'husband', 'brother', 'uncle', 'grandfather', 'mate', 'worker'. In other words, the *praxis* of father, husband, worker and so forth, is the principal 'means by which the individual's masculinity and health is socially affirmed'. To be both male and 'functionally fit' for one's social roles and responsibilities, from this perspective, is itself a measure of the degree to which one has 'social fit' (2000: 119). 'Being in shape', in this respect, is more about the need to fulfil the demands of pragmatic everyday embodiment than the actual shape of the body according to normative standards, stereotypes or ideals. Men often spoke about the *perceived restrictions on time that work, marriage, fatherhood involved, and the 'sacrifices' this entailed*, particularly as far the cultivation of the physical body and engagement in 'healthy' practices were concerned.

Sleep, it may be ventured, fits more or less readily into the picture here. Being 'socially fit' for one's roles of worker, husband, father and so on, may also involve varying degrees of 'sacrifice' as far as men's sleeping as well as waking lives are concerned, particularly *if* or *when* they embrace more 'egalitarian' ideals regarding children and the gender division of labour or 'second shift' (cf. Hochschild with Machung 1990)[14]. The UK 2000 Time Use Survey, in fact, finds that women on the whole sleep longer than men, particularly in the 30–60 age range (ONS, 2003). These aggregate figures themselves, of course, are far from unproblematic. They nonetheless introduce a further note of caution into the debate raising important questions about the nature and status of men's sleep. Women, then, *may* be disadvantaged as far as their 'right' to sleep is concerned, and women *may* experience more sleep disruption than men, but men's sleep may be compromised or disturbed in all sorts of ways too through their competing roles and responsibilities, at home and at work, lived and enacted through pragmatic modes of embodiment in everyday/every night life. Men, indeed, may report equally important cases of compromised or disturbed sleep. The result, harking back to Popay's (1990) study, may well be different types of tiredness, but the influence of different types of masculinity on the very 'doing' of sleeping, including talk about sleep-related matters, weighs heavily in any such balance sheet.

Ageing and later life

As for questions of sleep in 'later life', the picture here too is complex and contingent if not contradictory. The architecture of sleep, recalling an earlier point, may well change as men and women 'age', but this itself, in keeping with the foregoing themes and issues, is accompanied by a series of changing roles and responsibilities, statuses and identities which also need accounting for. This may include the transition from 'work to retirement, from good to poor health, from an active to a more sedentary lifestyle, from caring for children to caring for elderly parents or a spouse, and from spouse to widow(er)' (Hislop and Arber 2003b: 189). As lives and lifestyles are 'restructured', so too are our sleep patterns, with 'earlier expectations and patterning of sleep no longer viable as roles undergo change' (2003b: 189). The life course may itself be seen, in part at least, in terms of the structuring, unstructuring and restructuring (or doing, undoing and redoing) of sleeping, according to changing roles, relationships and responsibilities. To repeat, we may well then experience more 'fragmented' (and lark-like) sleep as we get older, and we may well suffer an increasing number of ailments or health problems, which themselves of course compromise the sleep of sufferers and partners alike, but these very factors mesh in complex ways with many other facets and features of our social lives and relationships as we 'age'. Our sleep therefore is the 'outcome of the interaction of life events in association with the physiological ageing of both the mechanisms of sleep and the body' (2003b: 189; see also Morgan 1987 for a similar interactive viewpoint[15]). These factors, in turn, interact in gendered ways to produce a 'fertile environment for the emergence of compromised sleep patterns as individuals age' (2003b: 189).

Financial hardship may be another important factor as far as sleep is concerned, particularly for women in later life (Arber and Ginn 1995). Poverty and hardship, as Morgan (1987: 68) notes, may compromise sleep in all sorts of ways, from hunger through inadequate diet, to inadequate beds and bedding and poorly heated housing during the cold winter months. The likelihood of spending even a brief period of time in some form of institutional setting also steadily increases with age, which again may negatively impact upon the quality of sleep in numerous ways, including the initial strangeness of a new setting or environment, its psychological impact, or its 'sheer disregard for peace and quiet!' (1987: 70).

Caution is needed, however, lest an overly negative or problem-centred picture of decline or disadvantage in later life, sleep-related or otherwise, is painted here. Other currents within the sociology of ageing, for instance, whilst admittedly not addressing sleep-related matters, paint a more positive picture of later life, suggesting that ageing in late/postmodernity is being increasingly 'destabilized' as less and less emphasis is placed on age-specific role transitions or scheduled identity developments and more 'fluid', 'active' forms of ageing come to the fore. There are many options for 'doing' and 'undoing' ageing, particularly amongst those with sufficient resources. It is indeed, we are told, this very fragmentation of a 'highly socialised biological process' (what Featherstone and Hepworth 1998 refer to as 'bio-cultural destabilisation'), which makes ageing such a key or critical feature of our times (Gilleard and Higgs 2000: 1). Ageing then, from this perspective, cannot solely or simply be equated with decline or disadvantage. On the contrary, a variety of possibilities have opened up which in turn link the (un)doing of ageing and gender with the (un)doing of sleeping.

It is not necessarily a question of choosing between these viewpoints, however, but of reconciling them. Bury's (2000) comments, for instance, are instructive on this count. Sociological concepts of 'biographical *continuity*' and 'biographical *disruption*' across the life course, he argues, which *combine* the influence of *disadvantage* with a recognition of the possibilities of significant *positive* changes in social relations, hold out the prospect of a 'fruitful sociological focus'. The 'biographical relays' between 'continuity and change', constitute a 'major vantage point for future medical sociological research on health, ageing and the life course' (2000: 102–3). The same might be said of sleep, or the (un)doing and redoing of sleeping across the life course, in which issues of continuity and change, both positive and negative, loom large. Far from mere 'time out', sleep is an integral part of our biographies, disrupted or otherwise.

From here it is but a short step to related questions of sleep and intimacy.

To share or not to share? Sleep, sex and intimacy

Earlier the point was raised that the 'doing' or 'undoing' of sleeping was not simply a question of *when* one sleeps or *how* one sleeps, but of *where* and with *whom* one sleeps. Historically, as we have seen, it may have been common practice to share a bed or sleeping space with all manner of people within and beyond one's immediate family circle, but the privatisation or sequestration of sleep gradually raised the threshold of shame and feelings of intimacy and taboo regarding such practices, restricting them to our nearest and dearest. To share or not to share, in this respect, raises a host of issues which themselves are negotiated in an ongoing fashion within couples and families. Doing sleeping and doing intimacy, from this perspective, are themselves intimately related.

Take co-sleeping practices amongst parents and young children for example. This, it seems, is a common practice around the world, even in

Western cultures today (Lozoff 1995). Many parents in the West, whatever professionals might think or say, sleep with their young children. Some degree of co-sleeping, for example, has been noted in approximately half of families with young children, with significant class and ethnic relations: that is, a greater prevalence of such practices amongst lower social classes and ethnic minority groups (Lozoff 1995: 71). 'Separation' and 'autonomy', in this respect, may be legitimate (Western) concerns, but the emotional warmth and comfort that co-sleeping brings is considered important in family life, particularly where young children are concerned.

As for the doing of sleeping and intimacy amongst adults, a number of points are worthy of comment. First, sexual relations themselves, particularly *illicit* or *extra-marital affairs*, are frequently referred to or dressed up through the discourse of dormancy. 'She is sleeping with him', 'he is sleeping with her', 'they are sleeping together', are commonly heard refrains, whether or not any sleeping occurs! To 'spend the night together' or to 'bed' someone are further interesting variants on these themes. To actually sleep with someone, however, denotes a level of intimacy over and above the purely physical, carnal or sexual act. The sexual intercourse that precedes or follows sleep, in this respect, constitutes only one aspect of intimacy if not infidelity (Schwartz 1970: 494). 'The lover's decision to share a single location', in other words, 'lifts the relationship beyond the purely physical and stamps it with an intimacy that cannot be claimed when the termination of the social relationship coincides with the termination of its sexual component' (1970: 494). 'We only slept together' may be a mitigating clause here, as far as the accused in an illicit or extra-marital affair is concerned, but either way, the intimacy of sleep cannot be denied. Nor can the damage, for ongoing coupledom, of sleeping 'under another roof' (Schwartz 1970), in 'another's bed' or 'playing away from home'.

We may also ponder further the literal as well as metaphorical links between sleep and sex. Whilst sleeping with someone, as already noted, may very well denote a level of intimacy and a shared bodily vulnerability over and above anything remotely sexual, both sleep and sex may be (intensely) pleasurable 'releases' involving a relinquishing of rational control, a loss of self (containment), and an immersion in the more carnal or sensual aspects of our embodiment[16]. Sleep, in this sense, recalling Rabelaisian carnival culture (Bakhtin 1968) and Bataillean themes of the erotic and the excessive (Bataille 1987/1962), harbours its own transgressive possibilities, including of course the pleasure of erotic dreams as well as the horrors of the nightmare (see also Chapter 1 on dreams and Chapter 2 on the carnivalesque/transgressive nature of 'indiscriminately mixed' sleeping bodies of past centuries[17]).

The second issue, building on these preliminary insights and speculations, concerns the doing of intimacy through sleep within ongoing coupled relationships. The actual act of sleeping together may involve companionship, intimacy, mutual trust and vulnerability – to say nothing of the comfort of somebody beside you when you awake with a start in the night – but pre- and post-sleep bed-bound practices may also prove an important part of coupledom. 'Pillow talk', for example, may be a valued and valuable part of relationships. Research by the Sleep Council (2002), for instance, found that for the majority of couples studied these night-time chats whilst snuggled up in bed together kept their 'romance fresh' and the 'love alive'. Nearly six out of ten couples (58%), in fact, confessed to revealing their most 'intimate secrets' to one another during pillow talk, compared to one in five (19%) who engaged in such deeply personal exchanges whilst out walking and one in ten (9%) who swapped secrets over the breakfast table. Women, unsurprisingly perhaps, were more likely than men (63% against 54%) to value and enjoy pillow talk, as were younger couples. Eight out of ten (80%) of younger couples chatted away in bed together compared to just four in ten (41%) of the over-55s – the latter, in contrast, were more likely to talk over the breakfast table or when out walking (Sleep Council 2002). Whether or not, of course, sleep is 'the new sex' (Demetrious 2004), where incompatibility of sleeping partners leads to relationship breakdown, is a moot point. Either way, the relationship between the doing of sleeping and the doing of intimacy is clearly an important one with which all couples, new or long-standing, must contend.

There is also, of course, the symbolic significance of sharing a bed as an indicator of the nature or current state of the relationship. To sleep apart in separate rooms, rightly or wrongly, is often considered a blow to the relationship, and to permanently do so at least a sign that the 'rot has set in'. This may or may not be the case, but the impression lingers and may necessitate a redoubling of effort on the couple's part. These perceptions, however, do depend on the length of the relationship. The aforementioned Sleep Council study, for instance, found that fewer than half (45%) of those who had lived together for less than five years were worried about causing offence by suggesting separate beds, compared to two thirds (62%) of couples whose relationships had lasted six years or more.

Further insights into these issues are again provided in Hislop and Arber's (2003a) work on gender, sleep and ageing. They note that the expenditure of emotional labour, echoing previous themes, may also extend to the partner with whom a woman shares her sleeping space. Concern for her partner's well-being, in this respect, may include responsibility for his sleeping as well as his waking life, including feelings of guilt if she disturbs his sleep. On the other hand, having a snoring partner is commonly blamed for women's own sleep disruption. For one woman, for example, her husband was transformed into an alien-like unhuman figure through his terrible snoring:

> (My husband's) one of those people who can go to bed quite happily at
> 10pm, so by the time I come stumbling upstairs, *it* is sort of a snoring
> heap.
>
> (Hislop and Arber 2003a: 704)

The stigma of snoring, of course, or perhaps more correctly the stigmatising consequences of being labelled 'a snorer' (cf. Goffman 1981/1963), is
itself likely to be heavily gendered and more of a problem for women than
for men given prevailing notions of masculinity and femininity[18]. Issues of
(in)considerateness, (in)sensitivity, if not (ir)responsibility, also arise here.
Can the snorer, for example, be held accountable for his or her snoring?
Well, yes and no. No, to the extent that snoring is an involuntary act, of
which the snorer is blissfully unware. Yes, to the extent that steps can be
taken to alleviate if not remedy the problem, with or without the aid of the
sleep clinic. If a snorer persists in doing nothing about their snoring, despite
frequent complaints from their long-suffering partner, an element of
blameworthiness or culpability creeps in through the back door, so to speak.

This begs another gendered sleep question: are men more 'selfish' or
'inconsiderate' sleepers than women? Findings from Hislop and Arber's
study certainly seem to suggest so. Men, it appears, may act in a manner
which shows a lack of sensitivity that 'blatantly compromises their partner's
access to the sleep resource' (2003a: 704). For many women the bedroom
resembled something like a 'battleground' in which partners engaged in a
'power struggle for sleeping rights':

> If my husband has got a problem and he is sort of waking up at 3 or 4
> o'clock you know he will say, 'are you awake?', as though he is trying
> to get through to me. And I say 'well I am awake now' and he says
> 'well, can we talk now?' And he will put the light on.
>
> (quoted in Hislop and Arber 2003a: 704)

Embedded in this is a further potential struggle between dark and light as
regards pre-sleep rituals and routines. My partner, for example, likes to
read in bed with the light on. I, however, like to dive into bed and switch
the light off immediately. On good days (or nights) we can coordinate this
quite well. She will go off to bed earlier than me to get her reading time in
before I hit the sack, at which point lights happily go out with the consent
of both parties. On bad days, however, this arrangement sadly breaks down
and a tussle duly ensues, with me sleeping with the light on, or her plunged
into darkness before a page is turned.

Partners, as this suggests, may act as 'gatekeepers' to each other's sleep
qua right or resource, which itself, in keeping with Hislop and Arber's
(2003a) general line of argument, reflects gender inequalities. Sleep
disturbance or disruption, in other words, may well be an important yet

'invisible' part of the pleasures and pains of partnership or coupledom – from partner's snoring, tossing and turning, to hogging the bed clothes, nocturnal chats, reading, watching TV or listening to the radio (Sleep Council 2002) – but women it appears are far from equal partners as far as sleep as a resource and a right is concerned.

Here we return to the question of *strategies* in the face of sleep disruption, and the tricky issue of whether or not to 'relocate' on a temporary or permanent basis; the symbolic connotations or (stigmatising) consequences of which, to repeat, can be problematic for couples, particularly those in long-term relationships. Whilst many couples still sleep in the same bed, regardless of the degree of disturbance they face, an increasing number of people are choosing to 'vacate' the double bed and debunk the symbolic baggage that goes with it in favour of a good night's sleep elsewhere (Hislop and Arber 2003a,b; Sleep Council 2002). As far as permanent sleeping relocation is concerned, for example, a number of women in Hislop and Arber's study questioned the tradition of having one bed for the dual purpose of sex and sleep, believing that 'better sleep and greater harmony can be achieved by having separate rooms *without jeopardizing the quality of the relationship*' (2003a: 707). One's sex life, moreover, may actually be *enhanced* through such a strategy. A recent article in *The Guardian* (Radice 2003) posed the question of whether or not couples who sleep apart can really stay together, and whether or not it is possible to maintain a sex life if you sleep apart. It reported the case of a couple who have tried to sleep together for the past 15 years with varying degrees of success due to a snoring husband. The report states that the wife used to decamp to the sofa bed as and when required during the night, but in the past year has given up trying to sleep with her husband and simply started the night on the sofa bed. Their sex life, however, has improved no end since sleeping apart. 'I have been amazed', she tells us, 'we have more sex now, but in my study because maybe it is more exciting. It is our sexroom now and there is a frisson that wasn't there before' (quoted in Radice 2003: 7).

Temporary, intermittent, or 'contingency' relocation is another option, of course, when the ability to 'put up' with disruptions associated with one's partner's sleep on occasion proves 'too much' (Hislop and Arber 2003a). The ability to do so, however, is of course dependent on the sleeping space options available for the partners in question, which may reflect material circumstances as well as their point in the life course. By the time children leave home, for instance, space may be less of an issue, particularly for those in working-class households. Whether permanent or temporary, nonetheless, relocation may also engender a variety of emotions, including guilt or anger, resentment or frustration, on the part of the 'deserter' and the 'deserted' alike.

It is not simply a matter of troublesome partners and temporary or permanent relocation strategies, however. Bereavement, separation and divorce may also significantly affect sleep patterns, for better or worse. Divorce in later life, Hislop and Arber (2003b: 197) note, can bring a sense of 'freedom' to some women and, after an initial period of mourning the relationship, often an 'improvement in sleep patterns'. For many people, nonetheless, the 'empty double bed', whether through separation, divorce or death, is a 'constant reminder of the couple relationship that was' (2003b: 197), and an expression of their newfound (unwelcome or unwanted) identity as single, 'dumped', bereaved or divorced. It may also engender newfound feelings of insecurity and vulnerability as the lights go out and one is left to face the dark, that terrible incapacitating existential darkness, on one's own.

To summarise, this penultimate section amply testifies that sleep is frequently 'done' and 'undone' together, by couples and with children and families across the life course. The double bed indeed may be the site of our most intimate moments, a 'comfort zone' predicated on the mutual sharing of our secrets and vulnerabilities, but it may also prove something of a 'danger zone' or 'battleground' where gender inequalities are writ large. Strategies of sleep relocation, in this respect, whether permanent or temporary, must contend with the symbolic and emotional significance of sleeping apart, and may or may not improve your sex life! However, it is surely the act of *'sleeping together'* rather than sleeping with 'men' as such, as Crossley (2004) rightly observes, that generates a 'politics of sleep'. Sleeping together, by virtue of the mutual consideration it requires, is a 'form of interaction which generates interdependency, which in turn constitutes a power ratio and thus "politics" of sleep' (2004: 23), or perhaps more correctly a micro-politics of sleep. Lesbian and gay couples, in this respect, may experience 'a very similar sleep politics' (2004: 23): a contention which itself clearly warrants further research. Sleep and domestic violence – what could be considered the 'dark side' of the politics of sleep – is an issue we shall return to and consider more fully in Chapter 4.

Sleep, liminality and death

From these considerations of sleep, sex and intimacy, one may tip-toe on to related matters of sleep, liminality and death. It would, of course, be crass to claim any simple or unproblematic equation of sleep with death or dying. Sleep, recalling issues first aired in Chapter 1, is a reversible loss of consciousness of the waking world; death is not, save for those lucky few who are 'brought back' from (the brink of) death through a (medical) miracle of one kind or another.

There are, nonetheless, some instructive parallels between sleep, death and dying. Sleep, as previously noted, is a 'liminal state' somewhere between wakefulness and death. There are, moreover, a series of 'intermediate positions' between 'deep sleep' and fully alert wakefulness. Death and dying too, depending on custom, culture and convention, may be regarded as more or less extended periods of liminality, particularly when visions of the 'after life' and the modern-day Western transition from 'quick' to 'slow', if not 'dirty', dying are taken into account (cf. Lawton 2000). In both cases, the conscious demands of the waking world are relinquished, temporarily or irrevocably. We also, of course, not infrequently, die in our sleep: what many think of as a merciful release or most peaceful way to go.

The links between sleep and death, in fact, can be traced way back to ancient Greek mythology where Nyx, the goddess of night, gave birth to Hypnos (the god of sleep) and Thanatos (the god of death). Poets too, such as Donne, Bunyon, Coleridge and Shelley, have waxed lyrical about the blessings of sleep and his 'brother' death: 'both so passing, strange and wonderful!', in Shelley's immortal words[19]. Notions such as the 'Big sleep' and 'Rest in peace' (RIP) likewise abound in lay and popular culture: attempts perhaps to civilize, soften or tame the 'finality' if not 'obscenity' of death. Sleep, without wishing to push these analogies too far, may even be something of a 'dress rehearsal' for death: a substitution, borrowing from Bauman (1992), of 'reversible' death and temporary disappearance for the irrevocable termination of life itself.

This perhaps is a fitting place to stop, lest sound or solid points give way to pure speculation. There is a world of difference, in short, between dormancy and death, let alone dying, but this should not blind us to fruitful comparisons and contrasts stuck, both historically and cross-culturally, between these twins of mother night.

Conclusions

Where then does this leave us?

The leitmotif or integrating theme of this chapter, it is clear, is *embodiment*: an extension, in effect, of former embodied concerns to this 'dormant' third of our lives. Phenomenologically, as we have seen, sleep involves a more or less radical alteration in our conscious, temporal relations with the waking world – a transition, that is to say, from an 'ecstatic' to a 'recessive' mode of embodiment or 'depth disappearance' in which the body is recessed from my conscious awareness, command and control (cf. Leder 1990). Sleep, we might say, with the notable exception of dreams, is an embodied non-experience which is *liminal* in at least two principal ways: first because it is inferred rather than directly experienced; second, because it is neither an entirely voluntary or involuntary, purposive or non-purposive phenomenon. As a rapidly reversible state, furthermore, our loss of consciousness to the outside world is far from total. The sleeper, to repeat, is never completely severed from the intersubjective world *qua* sleeper. Beyond deep sleep and alert wakefulness, moreover, lie a range of intermediate states which underline this liminal point of view.

Sleep is not simply *embodied*, however, it is *embedded* in the social world: embodied and embedded, that is to say, in a network of social roles and relations (cf. Crossley 2004). The (un)doing of sleeping, as we have seen, sheds further sociological light on these issues, alerting us to the *methods*, *motives*, *meanings* and *management* of sleep everyday/everynight life (Taylor 1993), including the role of (reflexive) body techniques that bring sleep under our own albeit *partial* control as embodied agents. Our biological or physiological need to sleep, in this respect, may well mean that we pursue our social projects 'on a leash', so to speak, but we still have con-siderable discretion over when, how, and where we sleep. To the extent that we may meaningfully talk of a sleep role in this context, it is clear that this, shorn of Parsonian (consensual) assumptions and fixed role prescriptions, involves a reciprocity of rights and responsibilities on part of the sleeper and significant others, which themselves are (re)negotiated in an ongoing, contingent fashion (cf. Crossley 2004). The *legitimacy* of sleep, in turn, depends on the context and the circumstances in question. Relations between the biological and social state of sleep, in this respect, are complex and contingent, including the intriguing notion of the 'socially attentive' sleeper.

Life course issues and biographical themes of *continuity* and *change* mesh closely with these matters, adding further embodied insights regarding the (un)doing of sleeping from childhood to (deep) old age. A fuller more dynamic picture of sleep begins to emerge at this point: one in which phys-ical, psychological, social, cultural and economic factors intertwine in complex *gendered* ways across the life course, including changing roles, relationships, responsibilities and critical life events. Sleep 'disturbance' or 'disruption', from this perspective, may be a more or less 'normal' part of the life course, depending on circumstances and situation: a process one might say of doing, undoing and redoing sleeping throughout our lives, suc-cessfully or otherwise. Moreover, our biographies do not simply begin and end with our conscious waking selves: we are sleeping as well as waking beings unto death.

The (un)doing of sleeping and the (un)doing of intimacy are also, it is clear, closely interrelated. From illicit sexual liaisons and co-sleeping pat-terns and practices amongst parents and (young) children, to the ups and downs of embodied and embedded coupledom, the pleasures and pains of sleeping together provide yet another 'window' onto the world of intimate relations and gender inequalities. To the extent that sleep, like sex, is a pleasurable 'release' involving a relinquishing of rational control, if not an immersion in the erotic or the excessive, then it too displays important elements of corporeal transgression.

As for the gendered politics of sleep, women may be more disadvantaged than men as far as the right to sleep is concerned, and much physical and emotional labour may go into caring for and managing the sleep of one's nearest and dearest, but we should not lose sight of the sacrifices and compromises which men also make regarding their (right to) sleep in their roles as workers, fathers and so on. Different types of masculinities, in turn, may impact on sleep in variable ways within and beyond coupledom or fatherhood. It is sleeping together, which, in all likelihood, generates a 'politics' of sleep (Crossley 2004).

Finally, a variety of literal and metaphorical links can also be traced between sleep and death, from Ancient Greek mythology to dying in our sleep. Whether or not sleep is a 'rehearsal' of or for death, a miniature reversible or revisable 'death', is a moot point, but a provocative note to end upon nonetheless.

Notes

1 This, of course, is not to deny the learnt, purposive or reflexive elements of sleep or sleeping, of which more later.
2 There are elements of Sartre's *Sketch for a Theory of the Emotions* (2001/1939) perhaps, *mutatis mutandis*, that are applicable here too. Certainly sleep may be construed in Sartrean terms as something akin to a 'magical transformation' of our being-in-the-world if not an 'escape' from it. Whilst Sartre is frequently criticised for wittingly or unwittingly reinforcing the commonly held view that emotions are 'irrational', 'regressive' modes of being or existence, this seems less contentious in relation to sleep given the loss of waking consciousness involved.
3 Schutz's take on the life-world runs as follows: 'In relation to other provinces of reality with finite meaning structure, the everday life-world is the *primary reality*. . .the life-world is the province of my *live corporeality*; it offers opposition and it requires exertion to overcome it. Everyday reality introduces me to tasks, and I must realize my plans within it' (Schutz with Luckman 1974/1973: 35).
4 Cases such as doctors legitimately sleeping whilst 'on-call', for instance, add further complexities here; see Chapter 4.
5 Thanks to Nick Crossley for extensive discussion of these issues.
6 Thanks to Bryan S. Turner for suggesting this apposite terminology.
7 Researchers are now, in fact, able to identify whether people, genetically speaking, have a lark or owl-like sleep propensity thanks to a difference in the CLOCK gene (Martin 2003). At the time of writing, the Science Museum in London is running a mass experiment to find out whether people are owls or larks through its 'live science' programme. Also see, for example, the following websites: http:// news.bbc.co.uk/1/hiprogrammes/breakfast/3703940.stm; www.sciencemuseum.org. uk/lets_talk/livescience.asp and www.surrey.ac.uk/SBMS/lark-owl.
8 Brannen and O'Brien note that, for some sociologists of childhood, children have been 'conceptually constrained by, and substantively contained within, the social institutions of family and school, rendering invisible their relationship to the wider social world' (1996: 1). Rather than detach children from their family setting, however, we need to '*recontextualize* children within their families, to begin to prioritise their interests and perspectives, and to take account of the permeability of the boundaries between families and the outside world and the ways in which children negotiate these' (1996: 1).

9 We are all social *actors*, one might say, but our social *agency* (our ability to shape and transform our situation in more or less efficacious ways) expresses our broader structural positioning (see, for example, Archer 1995).

10 A recent National Sleep Foundation Poll (NSF 2004), for instance, which focused specifically on children (aged 10 years and under), found television to be a common feature of their sleep environment. School-aged children were most likely to have a television in their bedroom (43%); however, 30% of pre-school children, 18% of toddlers and 20% of infants also had televisions in their bedrooms. Moreover, children who got less sleep were more likely to spend two hours or more watching television at home compared to those who got more sleep.

11 Studies conducted at the University of Minnesota in the 1990s, for example, showed that by starting school an hour later (at 8:30am), teenagers average sleep time increased by 45 minutes per night. They were also more likely to arrive at school on time, feeling less sleepy and less depressed, with fewer sickness absences, compared to those at similar schools where the early start time was retained (see, for example, Epstein 1998).

12 Hochschild's study (with Machung 1990) appositely entitled *The Second Shift: Working Parents and the Revolution at Home*, paints a moving and compassionate picture of couples struggling to find the time and energy for jobs, children and marriage, identifying a major division in gender ideology between a traditional ideal of 'caring' and another more 'egalitarian' one. A split between these two ideals, she shows, appears to run not only between social classes, but also between partners in marriages and between 'two contending voices inside the same conscience' (Hochschild with Machung 1990: 188–9): one in which women seem to come off worst.

13 We should also, of course, recalling previous themes related to children and childhood, note the disruptive and distressing effects of such episodes or events on children's sleep as well, alongside the uncomfortable feelings if not stigma these incidents may engender, even within the safety of the family and the family home.

14 A recent study of '*Involved' Fathering and Child Well-being* by Welsh and colleagues (2004) identified a continuum of parental involvement and family well-being ranging from 'child-centred families', in which the parents were highly involved, held egalitarian ideals, and were part of a supportive and amicable relationship, to more 'adult-centred' families, which had increasingly uninvolved parents with few emotional and social resources at their disposal. See also Lupton and Barclay (1997) for a study of discourses and experiences of fatherhood.

15 The ageing process, in Morgan's terms, can influence sleep either *directly* or *indirectly*. Directly influenced changes are those associated with ageing of the *physiological mechanisms that regulate sleep*. Indirect influences are those that 'arise outside of the physiological "sleep system" but, by impinging upon it, can profoundly affect the distribution and structure of sleep' (1987: 20). These events, in turn, can be subdivided into those that originate in the *physical environment* (mainly inside the body, such as disease, pain, discomfort and normal senescent changes in those physiological systems *not* directly related to the control of sleep) and those originating in the *social environment* (mainly outside the body) such as bereavement, living alone, financial hardship and institutionalisation. It is important then to recognise that 'age-related disruptions do not always result from some immutable biological change but may result instead from some reversible environmental condition' (1987: 66).

16 Mention should also be made here – harking back to the historical themes of Chapters 1 and 2 – of the work of Dr Marie Stopes (1918) who, in her book *Married Love*, forcefully espouses her views on the relationship between sleep and sex. There is, she tells us 'an intimate, profound and quite direct relation between the power to sleep, naturally and refreshingly, and the harmonious release of the whole system in the preferred sex-act' (Ch. VI). Women, in this respect, all too often fared worse than men, given 'the prevalent failure on the part of men to effect orgasms for their wives at each congress', which she claimed was, in turn, 'a very common source of the sleeplessness and nervous diseases of so many married women'. See also Stopes (1956) in which she sets forth many of her views on sleep, including her belief that anyone needing an alarm clock should take more sleep and that the head of the bed should always point northwards, or southwards, due to the magnetic forces of the earth.

17 Thanks to Chris Shilling for drawing these connections to my attention.

18 The snorer, to repeat, may be unaware of their snoring whilst snoring, but may still be labelled by their nearest and dearest as a snorer: a 'secret' that, if shared in public, may be more or less embarrassing depending on the individual, but influenced by the gender of the person in question.

19 Shakespeare also, of course, made much of these linkages, particularly in tragedies such as *Hamlet*: 'To die – to sleep – To sleep! Perchance to dream' (Act III, Scene i). Will there, in other words, be dreams after death? This appears to weigh heavily on Hamlet's mind when contemplating the existential question: 'To be or not to be?'. The idea of death as sleep, Lott (1970) comments, was perfectly familiar to Shakespeare's audience at this time. The Bible also uses images such as 'sleep in the dust' to represent death. See also Gadamer (1996) on the associations between sleep and death.

Chapter 4

The social patterning and social organisation of sleep: inequalities, institutions and injustices

Introduction

Already we have glimpsed or touched upon issues to do with the social organisation and social patterning of sleep, particularly historically. In this chapter we take a closer look at these issues in terms of contemporary trends and developments. Both this and the subsequent chapter may be seen as different takes or stances on the fate or fortunes of sleep in a changing social world, and the claim-making surrounding it, with particular reference to inequalities, institutions and injustices in this chapter, and the colonisation/commercialisation of sleep in the next chapter. Herein lies the rationale then for the remaining part of this book, which bring us right up to date, so to speak, in a long-running saga of sleep and society.

Our starting point, fittingly enough, is the (chronic) sleep deprivation debate and the broader questions of sleep and social change this raises: issues, as we shall see, around which much claim-making and a variety of interests compete or coalesce.

Sleep and social change: are we (chronically) sleep deprived?

> *I have noted as something quite rare the sight of great persons who Remain so utterly unmoved when engaged in high enterprises and in affairs of some moment that they do not even cut short their sleep.*
> (Michel de Montaigne 'On Sleep', 1572).

In Chapter 2 the argument was presented (via Ekirch) that sleep patterns and practices have not simply changed through the centuries, but that the *quality* of our sleep may actually have improved over time, while its *quantity* may have diminished. Whether or not we are all now (chronically) sleep deprived, in this respect, is an intriguing question which itself has engendered much debate in recent years[1].

Certainly there is plenty of evidence to suggest so, although methodological problems in researching these issues and comparing studies, including the 'normalisation' of sleepiness within and between groups in the lay populace, should of course be borne in mind at all times[2]. For example, a sizeable proportion of American adults (37%), according to the National Sleep Foundation *2002: Sleep in America Poll* (NSF 2002), report that they are so sleepy during the day that it interferes with their daily activities at least a few days a month or more; 16% experience this level of daytime sleepiness a few days a week or more. As many as 47 million adults, the NSF estimates, may be 'putting themselves at risk of injury, health or behavioral problems' because they are 'not meeting their minimum sleep need in order to be fully alert the next day' (NSF 2002; see also NSF 2001, 2003). In an earlier NSF Gallup survey of *Sleepiness in America* (NSF 1997) 32% of adults scored a significant level of sleepiness on the Epworth Sleepiness Scale. Indeed, 36% of these adults believed feeling *very* sleepy in the afternoon was normal (NSF 1997). Evidence from other countries also gives cause for concern. Around one in four British adults, for example, are thought to be suffering from chronic lack of sleep (Browne 2000), and more than a fifth of UK adults say they have 'severe' daytime sleepiness (Leadbeater and Wilsdon 2003). Also, 21% of Poles report feeling 'moderately sleepy during the day' (Zeilinski et al 1998), whilst 17% of Finns report daytime sleepiness 'often' or 'always' (Hyppä and Kronholm 1987). As for sleep 'down under', excessive daytime sleepiness (EDS) was detected in 11% of Australian adults according to one study (Johns and Hocking 1997). Even at a conservative estimate then, Partinen and Hublin conclude, 'frequent or excessive (subjective) daytime sleepiness occurs in about between 10–15% of the population' (2000: 563). It is also clear, on the basis of currently available evidence, that this occurs 'more often in school-age children or young adults than in middle-aged adults, and more often in females than in males' (2000: 563). Results, however, are said to be 'contradictory in middle-aged and older adults' with no clear-cut picture emerging (2000: 563). As for the variability of these results, this, to repeat, can be mainly attributed to methodological differences in the definitions and measures used, but probably also reflects 'real differences in different populations' (2000: 563).

These figures are backed up by further historical evidence which suggests that levels of (excessive) daytime sleepiness have risen over the years and that, on average, each of us sleeps approximately one and a half hours less than people at the turn of the twentieth century (Bliwise 1996, Webb and Agnew 1975). Americans, for example, according to the NSF *2002: Sleep in America Poll*, sleep on average 6.9 hours during the week, rising to 7.5 hours at weekends. Only a third of American adults (37%), the NSF *2001: Sleep in America Poll* reveals, say they get at least the recommended eight hours or more of sleep during the week, and almost a third of adults (31%) say they get less than seven hours sleep per night during the week[3]. On the basis of these and other figures, Dement (with Vaughan 2000) claims that, on average, Americans are walking around with a sleep debt of between 25–30 hours. The picture of sleep time in other countries is also revealing. Blaxter (1990), for instance, in the Health and Lifestyle Survey – a study of 9,000 adults in England, Wales and Scotland in 1984/5 – finds the population 'almost evenly divided' between those who claimed to sleep for 7–8 hours per night, those who 'usually' slept for less, and those who 'usually' had longer hours[4]. In Poland the population clocks up 7.1 hours sleep on workday nights (Zeilinski et al 1998), whilst, according to one large survey, approximately two thirds of Japanese people report sleeping less than seven hours per night, and more than a quarter, less than six hours per night. The latter figure rises to half amongst Japanese high-school students on week nights (Ohida et al 2001). All in all then, it is claimed that this research:

> . . . leaves little doubt that most adults in the USA, UK and other industrialised nations get substantially less than eight hours sleep most nights of the week, and many get less than seven.
>
> (Martin 2003: 22)

Even if we accept these conclusions, which are far from clear-cut or uncontested[5], the question remains as to whether or not this really matters. Isn't the recommended eight hours of shut-eye per night pretty much a myth anyway? Certainly, when asked, many people think they are not getting enough sleep, due in no small part to busy lives and squeezed timetables. For example, 30% of the NSF *2002: Sleep in America Poll* respondents said they needed a minimum of eight hours per night in order not to feel sleepy the next day, whilst, according to a recent Demos-commissioned MORI poll, 39% of British adults say they 'do not get enough sleep' (Leadbeater 2004). This figure in turn varies according to factors such as age, occupation, employment status and family responsibilities[6]. A recent UK 'precious time' ICM poll for *The Observer* (Reeves 2003) also found that 52% of adults surveyed stated that they would rather have more sleep than more sex if they had another hour in bed. Laboratory and home-based studies show that most people, if left to their own devices (i.e. without external interference) sleep between eight and nine hours per night (Bonnet and Arnaud 1995; Webb and Agnew 1975), although others suggest the figure is more like 9.5–10 hours per night (Coren 1996). Laboratory studies, moreover, suggest that nocturnal sleep periods reduced by as little as 1.3 to 1.5 hours for one night result in reduced daytime alertness by as much as 32% as measured by the Multiple Sleep Latency Test (MSLT) (Bonnet and Arnaud 1995). In other words, even modest amounts of *daily sleep loss*:

> . . . accumulate as sleep debt that is manifest as an increased tendency to fall asleep and a reduced level of psychomotor performance. Although

most people can resist this tendency. . .the likelihood of a lapse in vigilance, a 'microsleep' or a longer sleep episode can become high. . .. In work environments where sustained attention is necessary for safety, the probability of an accident rises and falls along with the biological tendency to fall asleep.

(Mitler et al 2000: 581)

These facts and figures, however, are further complicated by research which indicates that 'long' sleepers (i.e. those who sleep daily for nine hours or more) as well as 'short' sleepers (i.e. six hours or less) have increased mortality risks (Kripke et al 1979; Wingard and Berkman 1983).

This suggests that the (chronic) sleep deprivation thesis is far from clear-cut. Nor is it immune from criticism (Kryger 1995). Individual sleep 'needs', for example, are known to vary and the 'problem' (if problem it is) of self-defined sleep 'deficit' or 'deprivation' may be as much as product of perception as it is of actual time spent asleep. Harrison and Horne (1995), for instance, raise a number of important points and objections here, including problems with the historical evidence of reductions in self-reported sleep duration. Most people are *not* in fact chronically sleep deprived, they argue, but have the capacity to take more sleep, in much the same way that we eat and drink in excess of our physiological needs. We may, in this sense, be 'lean' rather than 'fat' sleepers these days, but by Harrison and Horne's reckoning: (i) sleeping beyond one's 'norm' produces, at best, only marginal benefits for the majority of the population; (ii) the ability to extend one's sleep time is not itself hard evidence of the need for this extension; (iii) the social and environmental contexts of sleep allow for considerable *intra*-individual variation in sleep duration and structure; and (iv) without this bringing appreciable improvements in subjective well-being throughout the day, 'many people are unlikely to be persuaded easily about the benefits of changing their daily sleep/wake pattern in order to take more sleep' (1995: 901–2). If we add to this other pertinent sociological questions as to whether or not the 'sleep' discourse is in fact, *in part at least*, a cipher, metaphor or vehicle, call it what you will, for something else (such as frustration, stress, anxiety or inequality) then there are indeed, without wishing to throw the baby out with the bathwater, grounds for caution on the (chronic) sleep deprivation or 'sleep crisis' front[7].

Nonetheless, these voices of caution or dissent, important as they are, are drowned out by the chorus of cries that (chronic) sleep deprivation is a 'real', widespread and growing problem in so-called 24/7 society, the costs and consequences of which are still being counted (Coren 1996; Leadbeater 2004; Leadbeater and Wilsdon 2003; Martin 2003; Moore-Ede 1993). The institutional supports and functions of the aforementioned sleep role (see Chapter 3), from this perspective, may be 'unravelling' fast in the 24/7 era where the rules of night and day are effectively 'superimposed' 24 hours a day; hence the growing 'politics of sleep' (cf. Crossley 2004: 28). 'Poor sleep', it is argued, 'has a price', including 'the struggle of many millions to stay awake at home, in school, on the job – and on the road' (NSF, nd). Sleepiness is said to contribute to 'more than 100,000 police reported highway crashes, causing 71,000 injuries and 1,500 deaths each year in the US alone' (NSF, nd). The financial cost of sleep-related accidents in the USA, excluding lost productivity, medical illness or shortened lifespans, is reported to be in the region of $56 billion each year (Mitler et al 2000). This, however, we are told, is merely the tip of the iceberg. From the *Exxon Valdez* oil spill to increased risks of heart attacks and strokes, the Challenger space shuttle disaster to deficits in mood, memory and IQ scores, the Chernobyl catastrophe to impaired immunity and behavioural or emotional problems at home and at school, the finger indeed is now firmly pointed, rightly or wrongly, at the 'poorly slept' if not (chronically) 'sleep-deprived' society. Human resources professionals and policy makers, it is claimed, need to 'wake up to the danger of creating a "sleepless society"' (Leadbeater 2004). Sleepiness, as Coren puts it:

> . . .is a health hazard to individuals. It may also be a danger to the general public because of the probability that a sleepy individual might trigger a catastrophic accident. . .. Perhaps someday society will act to do something about sleepiness. It may even come to pass that someday the person who drives or goes to work sleepy will be viewed as reprehensible, dangerous or even criminally negligent as the person who drives or goes to work while drunk. If so, perhaps the rest of us can all sleep a little bit more soundly.
>
> (1996: 286–7)[8]

These are issues we shall return to later in various guises, both in this chapter and the next. Suffice it to say for present purposes, that sleep, rightly or wrongly, is seen to be the 'casualty' of profound social, economic and technological change over the past century or so. In the 24/7 era punishing work schedules, unremitting deadlines, long work hours, lengthy commutes to and from work, the mixed blessings of the technological/online revolution, together with greatly expanded leisure and entertainment opportunities, these and many other factors, it is argued, have served to 'rob' or 'deprive' us of our sleep, resulting in 'reduced productivity' and 'tension at home' (Leadbeater 2004; see also Chapter 2 in this book on 'night as frontier' and the 'incessant society' [Melbin 1989]). Moreover, in an economy where we are 'much more likely to use our mind than our muscles', getting a good night's sleep is 'vitally important' (Leadbeater 2004). We have, wittingly or not, created all sorts of reasons for not sleeping, or cutting down on our sleep in favour of other pursuits and pastimes, pleasurable or otherwise, in a world that 'never stops' (Martin 2003: 26–9).

This, in turn, raises important questions about the relationship between sleep, time and technology in the late or postmodern era. Ours is an age, according to cultural theorists such as Virilio (1986), predicated on the logic (or illogic) of ever increasing *acceleration* or *speed* (what he terms dromology): a relentless logic, in Virilio's view, which lies at the heart of the organisation and transformation of the contemporary social world. The finer points of Virilio's (hypermodern) arguments regarding the human consequences of dromology – including the 'disappearance' of geographical space, time, matter, movement and aesthetics – need not concern us here. They have, however, generated fierce debate in academic circles – see Armitage (2000), for example.

The *acceleration* thesis does have its more mainstream supporters and popular advocates, resonating with the contemporary experience of many people today, who feel that life is indeed 'speeding up'. This is the 'heyday of speed', the era of the 'nanosecond', Gleick (2000) boldly proclaims in his tellingly entitled book *Faster: The Acceleration of Just About Everything*. 'Unoccupied time is vanishing', he argues, there is a sense of 'tension about time', we believe we have 'too little of it', we are 'in a rush', we are 'making haste'. Marketers and technologists, in response:

> . . . anticipate your desires with fast ovens, quick playback, quick freezing, and fast credit. We bank the extra minutes that flow from these innovations, yet we feel impoverished and *we cut back* – on breakfast, on lunch, *on sleep*, on daydreams. The defining quality is haste.
>
> (2000: 11, my emphasis)

Sleep itself can now be turned into 'productive time' (of which more later). Marketers, for example, try to sell us tapes promising 'to help you make money while you sleep, burn fat while you sleep, or learn a foreign language while you sleep'. Set up your computer properly, moreover, and you can even 'download megabytes from the Internet while you sleep' (Gleick 2000: 121). As for the sleep deprivation thesis, the mere presence of an alarm clock, Gleick claims, 'implies sleep deprivation, and what bedroom lacks an alarm clock?' (2000: 122; see also Stopes' 1956 equation of alarm clocks with the need for more sleep).

Again one may wish to quibble with Gleick's analysis here: part of the hype he is meant to be analysing perhaps? It does, nonetheless, speak more or less readily to the predicament many of us find ourselves in today. At one and the same time, we need to appreciate voices both past and present against any such trends. Russell (2004/1933), for example, in his provocative book *In Praise of Idleness* argues the case for less work, more leisure and the merits of quiet contemplative thought, cool reflection and 'useless knowledge': an antidote, he thought, to the misplaced virtues of work in a world of maddening unreason. Recent years have also witnessed what is now described, hailed or touted as an emerging 'slow movement'; a riposte, of sorts, to the cult of speed and a world obsessed with going faster. Gleick, to be sure, touches on these developments, but many people nowadays, it seems, individually or collectively, are choosing to 'slow down' and/or refusing to accept the dictatorship of speed or the decree that faster is indisputably good or inherently better.

Honoré, for example, in his recent book *In Praise of Slow*, charts this newly emerging Slow Movement which, in fittingly laid back fashion, has 'no central headquarters or website, no single leader, no political party to carry its message' (2004: 17). What matters nonetheless, Honoré assures us, is that a growing minority, a sizeable one indeed, is now 'choosing slowness over speed'. Every 'act of deceleration', we are told, 'gives another push to the Slow Movement' (2004: 17). Like the anti-globalisation crowd, Slow activists are:

> ... forging links, building momentum, honing their philosophy through international conferences, the Internet and the media. Pro-Slow groups are springing up all over the place. Some, such as Slow Food, focus mainly on one sphere of life. Others make a broad case for the Slow philosophy. Among these are Japan's Sloth Club, the US-based Long Now Foundation and Europe's Society for the Deceleration of Time.
>
> (2004: 17)

The Slow Movement, moreover, has already given rise to spin-off groups:

> ... under the Slow Cities banner, more than sixty towns in Italy and beyond are striving to turn themselves into oases of calm. Bra is also the home of Slow Sex, a group dedicated to banishing haste from the bedroom. In the United States, the Petrini [Italian founder of Slow Food] doctrine has inspired a leading educator to launch a movement for 'Slow Schooling'.
>
> (2004: 18)

As for sleep, we may simply note, for the time being, that there is much debate nowadays about the merits of (power) napping, both on and off the job, and that this in turn is backed up by a variety of 'Pro-Sleep groups', from the World Napping Organization to other more commercial ventures such as the nationwide network of 'Siesta Salons' in Spain (Honoré 2004: 214; see also Wilson 2004 and Winterman 2004).

Sleep, in short, is variably constructed or represented as casualty and corrective or symptom and solution to life in the fast lane. The notion of sleeping cultures, however, alerts us to important variations in this pattern or picture, both past and present, across the globe.

Cultures of sleep/sleeping cultures

Much of the discussion so far in this book has had an implicit, if not explicit, Euro-North American focus if not bias. Sleeping patterns and practices, however, vary widely across cultures and societies. Mauss (1973/1934), for example, in his deliberations on body-techniques and their social and cultural variability, informs us that war taught him to sleep anywhere and that all sorts of different ways of sleeping are practised throughout the world; some people sleep with pillows, some without, some in beds, some on the floor, some close together in a ring, with or without a fire, whilst some, such as the Masai, are able to sleep on their feet. This also extends to other techniques of the body, such as rest. Members of certain societies, for instance, Mauss comments, take their rest in what, through Western eyes, appear 'very peculiar positions' indeed. The whole of Nilotic Africa and part of the Chad region all the way to Tanzania (formerly Tanganyika), moreover, is populated by men who '"rest" in fields like storks: some manage to rest on one foot with a pole, others lean on a stick' (1973/1934: 81).

Findings from the World Wide Sleep Survey (see www.neuronic.com) – a far from representative source admittedly – shed more up-to-date light on these issues. In North Kenya's Ciabra tribe, for example, husbands sleep with their sons, and wives sleep with their daughters. The Paraguayan Aches apparently sleep on mats, whilst the South Venezeulans favour hammocks. As for the Kung! in North West Botswana, they sleep on the ground. The Efe in Zaire, however, go one better and sleep on thinly strewn leaves.

One way of making sense of sleeping cultures is to approach these issues with the help of a simple typology developed by Steger and Brunt (2003). At least three different ways of organising sleep, in this respect, are discernible here. In 'monophasic sleep cultures' sleep is concentrated into one consolidated block or period of time with a 'widespread ideal of an eight-hour nocturnal sleep phase' (2003: 16). A 'biphasic' sleep pattern is evident in 'siesta cultures', which take a short afternoon snooze and a longer sleep during the night. In both cases, Steger and Brunt (2003: 16) comment, the sleep role is 'protected from social demands to a certain extent'. A third possibility is a 'polyphasic sleep pattern' that is characteristic of 'napping cultures'. People in napping cultures usually have their 'anchor sleep' at night, and take individual daytime naps *as* and *when* the social situation allows or permits: hence the term polyphasic. A 'high level of tolerance rather than a set time', therefore, 'protects their daytime sleep' (2003: 16). All these patterns of distributing sleep throughout the twenty-four hour period, these authors stress, have developed 'in and of their own right' (2003: 16).

The monophasic nocturnal sleep pattern, of course, is widely found if not treated as the 'norm' in Northern Europe and North America. Any such normative reference point however, as already noted, is open to doubt.

Historically speaking, as Chapter 2 attests, the monophasic sleep ideal is a rather recent arrival in Europe. Many Westerners take regular naps, but the individualisation and privatisation of sleep has generally meant that day-time sleep is discouraged or avoided, save for children, the sick, the elderly and the night- or shift-worker. The need to protect night-time sleep then, Steger and Brunt (2003: 17) suggest, is 'quite strong' in monophasic sleep cultures, with 'transition periods' (cf. Schwartz 1970 and Goffman 1961a, 1963, 1967) from the sleeping role to the waking role 'comparably long and elaborate'. Ideally, the bedroom has the sole or 'solemn purpose of providing quiet and intimacy for sleep and possibly sex' and social rules 'dictate not disturbing sleep hours' (Steger and Brunt 2003: 17).

Meanwhile, siesta cultures are characteristic of Spain and societies with 'Spanish cultural influences'. Climatic influences may seem the obvious reason for the adoption of this sleep pattern, yet as Steger and Brunt (2003: 17) rightly point out, the siesta is 'neither restricted to countries near the equator, as the example of China shows, nor is it a habit found everywhere in Southern regions'. Neighbouring Portugal, for instance, hardly adheres to a 'socially set time for afternoon napping', whereas Greece does. In siesta cultures, on the whole, there is far greater tolerance of late-night activities, since the siesta provides an important 'buffer zone'. The siesta, nonetheless, is at risk in the global age, given the move towards an 'international clock' which is no respecter of local customs, timetables or traditions (Steger and Brunt 2003: 18). Again, these processes are complex if not contradictory. It may well be, in fact, that what we are witnessing is a decline of the siesta in the *southern* hemisphere (where physical Fordist-type labour predominates) and an emergence of the workplace nap in the *north* (where cognitive labour prevails) (Baxter and Kroll-Smith 2005): an issue we shall return to shortly.

As for polyphasic sleeping cultures, these can be found in 'every continent and under different climatic and socio-economic conditions' (Steger and Brunt 2003: 18). The emphasis here is on *flexible* rather than fixed sleeping patterns and practices that are fitted into or around other social roles, duties, activities and obligations. With regard to napping cultures such as China and Japan, indeed, Steger and Brunt suggest that at least two kinds of daytime sleep can be distinguished: the first involving the separation of the sleeper from waking activities; the second involving what was previously described, in Chapter 3, as *inemuri*, in which the sleeper is 'present in a situation that is meant for something other than sleep' (2003: 18). Sleep, in this respect (recalling the likes of Goffman 1963), may be a *main* or *side*, *dominant* or *subordinate* involvement depending on the situation in question. Even in societies such as China, Japan and India, that exhibit a high degree of tolerance towards daytime as well as public sleep, however, there are 'many occasions when sleep during social activities is not allowed' (Steger and Brunt 2003: 19).

Sleep cultures then are complex if not contradictory, and attitudes towards sleep may themselves be ambivalent or ambiguous within as well as between societies. Moreover, whilst napping is increasingly popular in other countries around the world as an efficient, flexible way of organising sleep in a global age, the idea of *inemuri*, as such, has 'not yet become global' (Steger and Brunt 2003: 20). It would equally be a mistake, Steger and Brunt stress, to draw too hard and fast a set of lines between 'Asian' and 'Western' sleep cultures, as if they were somehow hermetically sealed off from one another. 'Japanese, Koreans or Indians', for instance, 'pick up relevant American and European research as quickly as they are taken up in their own home country. The reverse is also true' (2003: 15).

Further insights into these convergences, contrasts, complexities and contradictions, within and between sleeping cultures over time, come from a variety of sources. Richter's (2003) interpretation of *early* Chinese literature, for example, reveals a discrepancy between texts that regard sleep as a 'natural phenomenon' and texts that focus on 'the social implications of sleep'. Whilst the naturalist or cosmological perspectives taken in medical writings, for instance, result in an 'impartial treatment of human sleeping and waking', the political writings of Confucian, Mohist or Legalist Provenance are generally 'partial': 'they explicitly favour waking and disregard or even despise sleep as they view man in a social rather than cosmological perspective' (2003: 39). This in turn contrasts with the Daoist compilation *Master Zhuang*, where sleep is characterised as a *positive counter-conception* in both a literal and metaphorical sense: not in the sense of recommending sleep but in the sense of 'a refutation of society's claim to control and instrumentalize the individual' (2003: 39). Moreover, contra the Confucian, Mohist and, in part, Legalist praise of waking, there is only a *'relative distinction* between the states of waking, dreaming and sleeping in the *Zhuang*' (2003: 38, my emphasis). These texts, Richter notes, serve primarily 'rhetorical purposes'. They do not, in other words, necessarily tell us anything about people's *actual* sleeping behaviour in early China (2003: 37). China, as noted above, may certainly be characterised as a napping culture on this latter count, both past and present; a deeply embedded feature of Chinese culture it seems. Western visitors, indeed, are 'still puzzled by the sight of sleeping Chinese and there is hardly a book of prints on China that is without a photograph of one or more picturesque sleepers' (2003: 24).

The Chinese midday nap, nonetheless, has been the subject of intense scrutiny, discussion and debate in recent years. The fluctuating attitudes towards the practice of napping in contemporary China and the West, Li (2003) argues, reveal two views that seem to take 'opposite directions'. First, while the Chinese have moved from the tradition of taking naps to abolishing or downplaying them, Westerners have moved from disdaining or disregarding them to respecting and emphasising them. Second, while taking or not taking a nap has now become an *individual choice* for the

Chinese, in the West it has become a broader social concern, and, therefore, a matter of social policy (2003: 61). Modernisation, in Li's view, is an important explanatory factor here. For Westerners who have, for the most part, modernised their economy, their concern has begun to lean towards respecting higher human needs – many see the siesta as one of those needs. For the Chinese, on the other hand, who are still moving along their path towards modernisation, the abolition of nap-taking is a price to pay for the 'ticket to modernity'. The different attitudes towards siesta in China and the West have therefore, 'epitomised the gap between the people in these two areas, not only in term of their cultures, but also in terms of the level of economic development' (2003: 61–2)[9]. Apparently the lengthy discourse on the practice of midday naps has currently 'waned' in China, with no clear-cut winners or losers in this debate. It is probable, indeed, that 'nobody will tell you whether or not you can take a nap, but the hastened pace in contemporary Chinese life has left little room for the practice to be continued' (2003: 62). The twists and turns of the discourse since the 1980s, therefore, Li concludes, can profitably be viewed as a 'windsock of the political climate in China' (2003: 62).

Instructive parallels can be drawn here with the changing fate of sleep and napping in Japan. Japanese sleep patterns, and the rationale for them, Steger (2003a) notes, display both *continuities* and *ruptures*[10]. Despite attempts begun in the late nineteenth century to establish or propagate an eight-hour monophasic sleep regime, Japan, Steger insists, can still be categorised as a polyphasic or napping culture. Polyphasic sleep patterns, in other words, appear to be the 'patterns of choice in ancient and pre-modern societies as well as present-day, twenty-four hour economies' (2003a: 83). In recent years, indeed, 'more and more people – medical doctors as well as businessmen – are promoting taking short daytime naps on a regular basis, and they promise that this habit will boost your intelligence and ability to succeed' (2003a: 83). Japan, in this sense, may well be ahead of the game here: a 'back to the future' scenario or sleep-smart option for the global age.

It is crucial then to be alive to issues of continuity and change, convergence and divergence, *within* and *between* sleeping cultures over time, particularly in the era of globalisation. Cultural pre/proscriptions, customs and conventions are clearly as relevant to our sleeping as our waking lives, including discourses and debates on the merits of the (midday) nap in Asia and the West.

Sleeping on/off the job: work time, work ethics and work stress

Issues of sleep or napping, work and economic life have already been touched on in this chapter, but now we turn to look more closely at the relationship between (paid) work and sleep[11]. I shall confine the discussion primarily to issues of work and sleep in the contemporary Western world, without in any way discounting or discarding the importance of comparative work of the kind identified above, and look at the following questions. What is the nature of the relationship between work and sleep in the current era? How is this relationship played out in different types of work or occupations? Is sleep another hidden dimension of inequalities in the workplace? How, moreover, do these issues mesh with broader discourses and debates on work stress in late or postmodernity?

Work, of course, may be intrinsically rewarding, with many positive benefits in terms of income, status, social inclusion and the like. The negative effects of certain types of work or working environments, however, for understandable reasons perhaps, have been the subject of most research, discussion and debate, particularly in the context of changes in work and employment since the mid-1970s. Much of this has focused on various aspects or dimensions of health status, rather than sleep as such, but general answers to the above questions can be found in prevailing wisdom and current research evidence.

Sleep, it is argued, is still not taken seriously enough in terms of work and employment practices, and health and safety issues in the workplace. Modern-day work, so the argument goes, is all too often a 'macho' culture in which sleep is 'for wimps': a workplace 'attack' on sleep, in effect (Leadbeater and Wilsdon 2003). Even when sleep is considered or discussed in such contexts it is often treated as little more than a vehicle for the advancement of broader ideologies concerning work time and work ethics, as many 'how-to-be successful' in business books attest (cf. Steger 2003a). To go without sleep, in other words, is all too often treated as a sign of 'commitment to your corporation and career' (Leadbeater 2004: 12). Demanding jobs, a long-hours culture, work intensification, together with job insecurities and other pressures of modern-day working life, are all potential disrupters of the quantity and/or quality of our sleep. The UK, for example, has the longest average working week in the EU. The Americans work even longer hours, whilst Asia has the dubious honour of being the hardest working continent with the least well-paid workers (Taylor 2003). Technology, in this respect, does not appear to have delivered the promise that many workers in the Western world had hoped for: instead of liberating or freeing us from the shackles of unnecessary or unwanted work, we just seem to be doing more, faster.

Epidemiological studies, in turn, suggest that the prevalence of sleeping problems varies by occupation (Partinen and Hublin 2000). In one large-scale Scandinavian study of 40 occupations, for example, 18.9% of bus drivers complained of having 'rather or very much difficulty falling asleep' compared to 3.7% of male directors and 4.9% of male physicians. Disturbed nocturnal sleep was complained of most often by manual labourers (28.1%

waking up at least three times per night) and female cleaners (26.6%), compared to 1.6% of male physicians, 7.4% of female head nurses and 9.4% of female social workers (Partinen et al 1984). When it comes to self-reported perceptions of sleep need, however, a somewhat different picture emerges, with managers and white-collar workers, according to the previously mentioned MORI survey of British adults (Leadbeater 2004), more likely to feel they are 'not getting enough sleep'. Shift work, in particular, is bad news when it comes to sleep (Åckerstedt 1995, 2004). Some shift patterns, however, such as (permanent) night shifts, are worse than others, with evidence pointing to increased risks of circadian rhythm disorders, gastrointestinal disorders, heart disease and cancer amongst such workers. Shift workers, if current evidence is anything to go by, seem to be less healthy, happy and productive, and more prone to accidents (Martin 2003; Åckerstedt 2004). With over 26 million Americans and nearly 4 million Britons doing some kind of shift work, not to mention those workers in other parts of the world, this is of no small importance, without taking into account further complicating factors such as gender and the problems that combining paid work with family responsibilities may pose for women's sleep (see Doi and Minowa 2003, for example, and Chapter 3 in this book[12]).

These issues, echoing previous themes of sleep and social change, need to be contextualised within the supposed transition from 'Fordism' to 'neo-Fordism', 'post-Fordism' or 'flexible capitalism': the 'Brave New World of Work' in Beck's (2000) terms. Traditional ideas and the expectation of a 'fixed' job 'for life' in the Fordist era, have given way to a new era of 'flexibility' and 'change', the net effect, for critics like Sennett (1998), being the 'corrosion of character' in the absence of a life-long career or vocation and no longer-term vision. The image, icon or anti-hero here, contra the traditional Taylorist production-line worker, is the dynamic, multi-skilled all-singing all-dancing team worker, infinitely adaptable to change, both in the workplace and in relation to broader, global market dictates. These processes, furthermore, are allied to new management structures and systems – such as 'just-in-time-production' and 'total quality management' – that result in much tighter and tougher surveillance and regulation of production, facilitated and enhanced by the latest forms of technology, the ultimate goal being a boost in productivity and profit, thereby squeezing more and more out of already hard-pressed workers (Wainwright and Calnan 2002: 124). Corporate 'mergers' and 'takeovers', 'downsizing', the 're-engineering' of traditional industries, 'flexibility' and 'change', are the buzzwords of working life and working culture in the twenty-first century as leaner companies and corporations compete in the global marketplace (Wainwright and Calnan 2002: 124). The irony here, as Martin (1994, 2000) notes, is that this new logic of flexibility is itself quite inflexible; a sort of neo-Social Darwinist survival of fittest in which rigid folk or inflexible souls fall by the wayside in the rush or stampede for change.

The emergence of sleepiness or drowsiness as significant workplace risk fits more or less readily into the picture here. From growing concerns over the problems of sleep-related accidents in the transport industry (road, rail, aviation, marine) (Dinges 1995; Horne 1999), to the risk of sleepy doctors, particularly junior doctors in training (Åckerstedt et al 1990, British Medical Association 2002, Deary and Tait 1987, Firth-Cozens and Moss 1998, Lewis et al 2002, Richardson et al 1996), the lines of the these debates can be traced: another prime facet or feature of the (chronic) sleep deprivation debate. This has led to calls for ever tighter controls and regulations in order to ensure not simply worker health and safety but public safety in general. Agreement was reached in May 2000, for example, on the arrangements and timetable for British doctors in training to be included in the European Work Time Directive (EWTD), with an interim 58-hour maximum working week from August 2004 and an August 2009 deadline for a 48-hour maximum working week – which itself may be extended by another three years at 52 hours if exceptional circumstances apply (see, for example, British Medical Association 2004; Carvel 2004a,b; Carvel et al 2004; Pickersgill 2001). The notion of sleep deprivation as part and parcel of professional socialisation persists, nonetheless, in certain segments of the medical profession at least (Green 1995; Patton et al 2001): an important part of the educational process, it is claimed, which solidifies identity, promotes group cohesion and solidarity in the face of adversity, and prepares the neophyte for incumbency of a powerful and prestigious social role. When Coren, for example, posed the question as to why one still sees residents and interns working on an average of four to five hours of sleep a night to the dean of a major US medical school, he received the following (mythology-infused) answer:

> The only way to stuff this information into the young doctor is through long hours. Furthermore, the argument goes, this a toughening process by which the doctor learns to make decisions under stress. . ... Many doctors view the period of being on house staff as something like an epic journey that the medical student must make. It's the epic of Orpheus, Dante or Hercules all over again. . ... Now he has to pass through hell, and in this netherworld he will confront his own limitations, suffer pain, strive against adversity. In the end, the traveller emerges from the underworld, and he has evolved to a new level.
>
> (1996: 203–4)

It is not simply a question of long hours or the trials and tribulations of shift-work systems, however, but of related issues to do with work stress and its impact on sleep.

Work stress and sleep: a modern epidemic in the making?

The disruptive influence of stress of any kind on our sleep doubtless makes intuitive sense to us all, but how does this square with the research literature and evidence on work stress? Much of this research, as previously noted, has focused on the relationship between work stress and particular aspects or dimensions of health status such as cardiovascular risk, rather than sleep as such. Many of these studies, nonetheless, include data on sleep. The picture in this respect, unsurprisingly perhaps, is complex, depending on factors such as individual reactivity to stress, the relationship between (high) job demands and (low) job control, effort-reward imbalances, and so on (see, for example, Åckerstedt 2004 for a useful review of the stress-sleep relationship, and Marmot and Wilkinson 1999, Siegrist et al 1990, Karasek and Theorell 1990, Lazarus and Folkman 1984, for other research on stress, coping and health status[13]). Research, for instance, has shown that individuals who are 'over-involved' with their jobs, or those suffering 'burnout', are at great risk of insomnia (Åckerstedt 2004, Martin 2003; Partinen and Hublin 2000). Other recent work on teachers highlights the potentially important role which rumination plays in mediating the relationship between work and sleep: the more we ruminate about work, broadly speaking, the poorer our sleep (Cropley 2004). It may not be work demands as such that are important here, in this respect, but rather their effects on 'post-work unwinding' (Åckerstedt 2004). Whilst the effects of stress on the risk of insomnia, moreover, are well established, sleep itself seems to yield the same physiological changes as stress, thereby complicating the picture still further (Åckerstedt 2004).

These findings resonate with lay accounts of the health and behavioural effects of work stress. Wainwright and Calnan (2002), for example, in a small-scale qualitative investigation of workers' accounts of their experiences of work stress, found sleeplessness to be a commonly reported 'symptom', alongside a broad range of other physical, psychological and behavioural 'symptoms', from palpitations, sweating, stomach trouble and headaches, through anxiety, depression and anger, to smoking heavily, excessive alcohol consumption and a drop in work standards.

To these findings we may add other research on issues such as job insecurity and unemployment; a potent, if somewhat paradoxical form of work stress, given the absence of work it threatens or symbolises. A robust association, for example, is found between unemployment, or the anticipated threat of redundancy, and poor sleep (Brenner et al 1985, Matiasson et al 1990). In a longitudinal cohort study of sleep during economic recession in Finland (Hyppä et al 1997), for instance, prospectively unemployed persons suffered more from insomnia and used more prescription hypnotics than the continuously employed. The sleep quality of the general Finnish population did not drastically deteriorate during this severe recession period, however, except among these unemployed blue-collar workers. Sleep disruption itself, Martin (2003) speculates, might play a role in the pervasive link found between unemployment and ill health, given the effects poor sleep can have on things such as immunological functioning, cholesterol levels and so forth (see also Åckerstedt 2004).

These findings are instructive; however, caution is needed, sociologically speaking, when considering the nature and status of the work stress phenomenon or 'epidemic'. Work stress is the number 1 complaint amongst British workers, according to a recent Trades Union Congress survey (TUC, 2002)[14], but, as Wainwright and Calnan (2002) rightly note, it is a 'contradictory category': something we can all more or less readily appreciate and identify with as workers in advanced western industrialised societies, but the subject of much controversy and debate. 'Is work really more demanding and pressurised than at any previous point in human history,' these authors ask? 'Has work become harder or have workers become less resilient'? 'Why was there no "epidemic" of work stress', for instance, 'between the two World Wars when many people, fortunate enough to be in work, faced incredible physical and mental hardship, uncertainty and insecurity'? 'Why', moreover, 'do problems and antagonisms that previously led to industrial disputes and collective action, now so often result in individual consultations with the doctor or counsellor' (2002: v–vi)?

The so-called work stress 'epidemic', from this more critical stance, may very well be a response to changes in work that have occurred since the mid-1970s, particularly processes of job intensification from the mid-1980s onwards, but it is 'broader socio-cultural changes – the heightened awareness of physical and mental vulnerability, the culture of victimhood, the emergence of the therapeutic state – that account for experiences at work being interpreted through the medicalised prism of epidemic and disease' (2002; 161). Work stress, in short, may well be very 'real' for those who experience it, of that there is no doubt, but it is also very much a product or phenomenon of the times we live in: an individualised and historically specific response to adverse work conditions and an 'amorphous category' at that, which itself is capable of supporting quite diverse interpretations, explanations and solutions to the 'problem' (2002: 23–32; see also Newton et al 1995).

This casts further critical light on some of the previously discussed claims and assumptions regarding sleep and social, economic and technological change in general, and the relationship between work and (chronic) sleep deprivation in particular. A closer inspection of long-term historical time trends, for example, shows that the actual number of annual hours worked, per person employed, has fallen by half between 1870 and 1998. Since 1950 it has fallen by 24% (Gottlieb 2004). Other figures lend further support to this picture. In the middle of the nineteenth century, for instance, Wainwright and Calnan (2002: 130) report, London's fitters and turners worked an average of 58.5 hours per week, week in week out. By 1968, however, manual workers not only enjoyed two to three weeks paid annual leave, but their average working week had fallen by a third to 40 hours. A similar pattern can be found for all workers for which there is reliable evidence. These aggregate or average figures, of course, far from tell the whole story about the changing nature of work over time, within or between groups. Productivity has also dramatically increased during the twentieth century, so too, by all accounts, has job intensification since the mid-1980s: a broad trend, it seems, across most sectors and segments of the workforce. By any measure, nonetheless, the evidence that we are working increasingly long hours is less than convincing, historically speaking. When it comes to questions of whether we are better or worse off than workers of the past, indeed, Wainwright and Calnan conclude, the safest, if rather unsatisfactory answer, is that 'work is "better" in some respects and "worse" in others, and that the net gain or loss will vary from group to group if not from person to person' (2002: 124). Despite this apparent need for caution, generalised claims about historical changes in work persist.

None of this, to be sure, invalidates the contention that society is (chronically) sleep deprived or in some sort of 'crisis' over sleep. Expanding leisure and entertainment opportunities, for example, are seen as prime culprits in keeping us from our beds and depriving us of our sleep. It does, nevertheless, introduce a further note of caution into the debate as far as the underlying causes and consequences if not the very construction of this contested phenomenon are concerned. It may very well be, for instance, harking back to an earlier speculative point in this chapter, that the 'sleep' discourse is itself far from adequate. Are we all talking about sleep, in other words, because it is a convenient cipher or way of framing other things such as frustration, stress, anxiety or inequality[15]? This, in keeping with the work stress discourse and debate, begs further important questions about the interpretation of sleep 'problems', in whatever shape, sense or form, through the medicalised lens or prism of epidemic and disease: issues we shall explore more fully in the next chapter.

Sleep, efficiency and the (power) nap: 'putting sleep to work'

> PN (prior to the nap) and AN (after the nap) may replace AM and PM as the proper way to divide the workday. . . .. And maybe in the not too distant future there will be three parts to a workday – PN, AN & DN – as in During the Nap.
>
> (Anthony and Anthony 2001: 11, 23)

A return to the changing fate or fortunes of the nap is also appropriate at this point, given the drive for ever more 'efficient' or 'smart' ways to sleep in the Western workplace and beyond[16]. A number of companies and businesses in the 'monophasic' sleep world today are beginning to wake up to the merits of the workplace nap as an officially sanctioned rather than an unofficially snatched practice: a case, quite literally, of 'putting sleep to work' in order to get the 'most' if not the 'best' out of one's employees.

In the US, for example, companies such as Pepsi, IBM, Pizza Hut and Kodak now run courses in the art of taking a 15-minute (power) nap, whilst Deloitte Consultancy, in Pittsburgh, has installed 'napping rooms' or 'napnasiums' for the comfort of their employees (Wilson 2004, Winterman 2004). Weary New York workers too can now take a nap during the day in specially designed pods in the Empire State Building, courtesy of *MetroNaps* (Winterman 2004). The UK may not be far behind. Leadbeater and Wilsdon (2003), for example, in a trailer for the recent Demos report *'Dream On: Sleep in the 24/7 Society'* (Leadbeater 2004), make a strong case for lifting the 'taboo' on public sleeping. In a 'well-slept' society, they claim, 'we could expect to see the provision of sleeping rooms, or hammock bays, as standard in offices and elsewhere, supporting a culture of extended power naps'. We could even, they continue, citing approvingly the Berlin 'dormitorium' where people drop in for a quick nap, see the emergence of new sleep services such as 'EasySleep' (Leadbeater and Wilsdon 2003: 42). This, in fact, is already happening. Mail order company Freemans, for instance, has four relaxation rooms for call-centre staff, whilst advertising agency St Lukes has a 'chill-out room' where staff can relax and recharge their batteries. Other companies, however, have gone one or more steps further, offering their employees a fixed number of 'duvet days', alongside other fringe benefits, when they are too tired for work: the soporific equivalent of a sick note perhaps? We may well wonder about the (corporate) motives and merits of all this – is it just the latest form of exploitation perhaps? – but the drive for effective or efficient sleep as a boost to productivity and performance, both on and off the job, is now increasingly apparent, in certain (economic) sectors or segments of society at least.

These initiatives are supported by studies such as Anthony and Anthony's (2001) above-cited book *The Art of Napping at Work* (see also Anthony 1997)[17], and the work of chronobiologists such as Claudio Stampi, author of *Why We Nap* (1992) and a leading expert on sleep and alertness management strategies for industrial operations and situations involving space, marine, aviation and surface transport operations. Stampi; indeed, has been at the forefront of developments to perfect polyphasic ultra-short napping techniques to sustain alertness and performance, while requiring only limited sleep, in these round-the-clock operations. This work has been applied in a variety of occupational programmes, including a NASA-commissioned project to design and study ultra-short sleep strategies for emergencies in space missions.

Perhaps the best known of these ventures, however, concerns Stampi's work with solo sailors such as Ellen MacArthur – Stampi himself, in fact, has participated in two around the world races as a Whitbread skipper. To help MacArthur successfully negotiate the heavy demands of her solo sailing feat during the Vendée Globe 2000, and to maximize her performance whilst at sea, Stampi worked closely with MacArthur, enabling her to master the art of the 'catnap' between the intense action of racing a boat 24 hours a day. When interviewed shortly after successful completion of the race, Stampi revealed that on average MacArthur had slept 5.7 hours per day, with a total of 891 naps (averaging 9.4 per day) and an average nap time of 36 minutes. The longest period of uninterrupted sleep, indeed, was a mere 2.8 hours, whilst the longest time without any sleep was 18.5 hours. 'Cluster napping' – which involved taking a series of naps interrupted by brief 2–8 minute awakening to monitor boat performance – accounted for 77% of MacArthur's entire sleep. These feats of human endurance, nonetheless, have subsequently been trumped by MacArthur's own recent record-breaking solo circumnavigation of the globe in 71 days, 14 hours, 18 minutes and 33 seconds. MacArthur averaged 5.5 hours sleep per day on this gruelling trip, typically broken up into ten naps, a third taken during daylight hours (Sample 2005). The most tiring/taxing week, however, began on January 5th 2005 sailing around Cape Horn, after 40 days at sea, with an average of 3.9 hours per day, dropping to an all time low of 1.5 hours on January 6th in eight short naps. 'I am numb to tiredness', MacArthur proclaimed on January 7th in her race log, 'as my veins are filled with adrenaline and fear. My brain is so active I cannot switch off at all' (Sample 2005). MacArthur, to be sure, returned home a hero (and a dame), but her record as far as sleep is concerned may be a somewhat chequered one; reinforcing perhaps, in the public's mind, the equation of lack of sleep with acts of heroism, bravery and moral virtue.

The humble nap, then, might not be quite so humble after all. It is instead part and parcel of broader trends and debates to do with work time, work ethics and the drive for ever greater 'efficiency' in our sleeping as well as our waking life: a quest for 'ultra-short sleep', that is to say, that makes you 'smart' and helps you to 'get ahead', whatever the challenge (cf. Steger 2003a). These processes, however, as previously noted, are variable or uneven across the globe, depending on factors such as economic sector, stage of economic development and the socio-cultural context of change. In the US, for example, 'the blurred distinction of public and private time follows a redescription of drowsiness as a workplace risk, the expansion of project-organized mental labor, and research on the economic and health benefits of a short nap at work' (Baxter and Kroll-Smith 2005: 51). In countries such as China, Spain, Italy and Mexico, in contrast, 'the more Fordist the production process the less likely the traditional *Xiuixi* or siesta will survive' (2005: 21; see also Li 2003 and Steger 2003a).

Whether or not the workplace nap is a 'positive' step towards a 'post-Fordist utopia' of blurred borders and flexible working conditions, or a 'neo-Taylorist extension of class- and knowledge-based directives to the most private of activities' (Baxter and Kroll-Smith 2005: 52), is an open question at present. Elements of both explanations and more time, Baxter and Kroll-Smith rightly suggest, are required to 'make a full accounting of this evocative behaviour' (2005: 30). One thing is clear, nonetheless, that in the US and Northern European context at least:

> . . .the workplace nap highlights an increasingly ravenous work culture that encroaches on modern boundaries between work and home; a culture capable of transforming private non-productive acts like workplace naps into regulated, public time-space behaviors.
>
> (Baxter and Kroll-Smith 2005: 52)

To this, extending the analysis still further, we may add the napping politician. Whilst the life of a top-flight politician may not exactly be a 'well-slept' one, and whilst Mrs Thatcher's (in)famous ability to get by on precious little sleep has become something of a legend in political circles, many politicians in fact, both past and present, favour the nap. Churchill, for example, was a famous napper, so too, apparently, is President George W. Bush: one of his few policies, perhaps, one might wish to endorse. Steger (2003b) also reports an intriguing series of articles in the Japanese weekly *Shukan Hoseki* on parliamentarians dozing during public, observable, working situations. Again, the notion of *inemuri* is invoked here as an explanation for this phenomenon (see also Chapter 3 in this book). The parliamentary session as a 'ceremonial event', she argues, is considered 'more important than the actual work done there'. Similarly, the 'commitment to a job is judged by the time and effort spent on it rather than by the efficiency with which it is pursued' (2003b: 195). Thus, the Japanese habit of inemuri does not necessarily reveal a tendency towards 'laziness'. Rather, it is an 'informal structural feature of Japanese social life intended to ensure the performance of regular duties by offering a way of getting *away* within the framework of their duties' (2003b: 195).

In these and other ways the nap provides another important index of continuity and change, both inside and outside the workplace: the political-economy of sleep one might say. To nap or not to nap, that is the question!

Battling or combating sleep: military manoeuvres and technological tampering

Sleep and napping are not simply issues within the economic or political spheres, however; there are various military manoeuvres on this front as well, both past and present.

The strategic use of sleep deprivation as a 'weapon of war', for example, is an old military trick or tactic. Prolonged sleep deprivation indeed is known to have played a significant role in many battles, past and present. Martin (2003: 82–4), for instance, reminds us how lack of sleep, uncontrollable stress and starvation produced a 'lethal cocktail' for Hitler's troops during the Battle of Stalingrad in World War II. Not only did fighting drag on into the harsh Russian winter, Soviet commanders ordered night raids, aided and abetted by night flares, loud music, propaganda broadcasts and other around-the-clock activities, in part to induce exhaustion and break the spirits of enemy troops. Many German soldiers, in fact, died from this combination of exhaustion, stress, cold and lack of food, rather than from Russian bombs or bullets. Finally, in February 1943, the tired and broken remnants of the German army duly surrendered (see also Beevor 1998).

Sleep has always played its part in warfare, although it may not have been recognised as such. It is only recently, however, that it has been more or less thoroughly incorporated into the planning, logic and execution of military operations; a transformation, in effect, of 'common sense' into explicit military rules and regulations based on the latest technological 'know-how'. This, in turn, has spawned a whole new military vocabulary, including terms such as 'sleep management strategies', 'unit sleep plans', 'sleep description', or 'sleep management systems' (Ben-Ari 2003).

The US, unsurprisingly, has been at the forefront of these developments in recent years, with potential applications not simply for various combat scenarios, but for other kinds of military deployment and shift-work systems (see, for example, Walter Reid Army Institute of Research [WRAIR] 1997). 'There is nothing heroic about staying awake for prolonged periods of time', Colonel Belensky, lead sleep researcher at the WRAIR outside Washington DC, states. 'In fact', he continues, 'combat soliders who deprive themselves of sleep can cause missions to fail' (quoted in Fleming-Michael 2003: 39). Sleep deprived battle planners too, who frequently get less sleep than the soldiers in combat, can make poor decisions; an undesirable combination of poor decisions amongst soldiers based on poor plans passed to them by tired planners.

The military, in this respect, studies sleep with regard to *sustained* and *continuous* operations, both of which take their toll. During sustained operations, combat soldiers get less than four hours of sleep each night for days at a time, which is considered severe sleep deprivation. During continuous operations, soldiers get less than seven hours sleep each night. Sustained operations, however, can occur *simultaneously* with continuous operations, thereby complicating further the mixed-up sleep patterns of already sleep-deprived soldiers (Fleming-Michael 2003: 40).

To mitigate some of these effects during military operations, WRAIR has a team of physicians, physiologists and psychologists who study sleep for the Department of Defence. To help commanders determine the effects of sleep deprivation, moreover, WRAIR researchers have developed a watch that measures how much sleep a subject gets and indicates how well an individual is performing and will perform in future. The sleep watch will be incorporated into the Objective Force Warriors 'Scorpion' ensemble as part of the Warfighter Physiological Status Monitoring System being developed by the US Army Research Institute of Environmental Medicine at Natick Massachusetts (Fleming-Michael 2003: 40).

Researchers have also looked at stimulants to see if they are effective in keeping soldiers awake and able to make sound decisions. The WRAIR is also testing caffeine, d-amphetamine and Modafinil (Provigil) (the latter drug is used to treat narcoleptics and excessive daytime sleepiness [EDS]) to see which of the three stimulants produces the best results[18]. The bottom line with stimulants, Colonel Belenky states, is that 'they are short-term fixes at best. The real answer is to get adequate amounts of sleep and efficiently managed sleep' (quoted in Fleming-Michael 2003: 41).

Matters do not end here, however. The quest for the no-sleep soldier also includes the efforts of the US Defence Advanced Research Projects Agency (DARPA), which has a multi-tiered programme concerned with *eliminating* the need for sleep during operations. These projects range from tinkering with a soldier's brain using magnetic resonance, to analysing the neural circuits of birds that stay awake for days during migration. The hope in doing so is to stump or trump the body's need for sleep, at least *temporarily* (Onion 2003).

As for sleep-inducing compounds to circumvent the body's natural circadian rhythms, army researchers are active here too. The US Army Aeromedical Research Lab, for example, has begun testing Zaleplon, a new sleep-inducing compound, to see if its hangover effect is less than the effect of previously tested hypnotics. Napping, likewise, is being re-evaluated. Colonel Belenky's advice, for instance, is again instructive here: 'Naps are wonderful', he says, 'take the opportunity to sleep whenever you can' (quoted in Fleming-Michael 2003: 42).

In these and other ways, then, the modern-day soldier is quite literally being 'geared up' to the eyeballs with the latest technological devices, gadgetry and fixes, including those designed for the promotion of sleep and wakefulness. Modern day (US) soldiers, in this respect, may well be kitted out with: intra-section radios, multi-spectral camouflage, combat identification systems, ballistic armour, night-vision goggles, sleep watches, stimulants and hypnotics, global positioning systems, night aiming devices, laser protection and individual weapons systems. Cyborg visions spring to mind at this point. Ben-Ari (2003), for example, suggests that these very devices and developments, including sleep management systems, seek to combine or merge into unified military systems comprising 'soldiers' bodies and brains, the concrete military machines they operate and the information systems to which they belong' (2003: 121). Borrowing from the likes of Gray (2002) and Haraway (1990), the individual soldier, he suggests, becomes part of a 'formal weapons system' through systems analysis, social psychology, physiology, psychopharmacology, behavioural sociology, personnel management, computer-mediated systems and the like (Ben-Ari 2003: 121). The sleep of soldiers, in short, is part of a:

> . . .wider set of systems that seek to blur the lines between soldiers and their environment by enhancing their bodies in ways that link them to the work of the armed forces, to machines they operate and to the new technologies that make the destructive potential of the military a concern that lasts twenty-four hours a day.
>
> (2003: 123)

Sleep(less) in. . .

Another important set of issues, following on from these economic and military themes, concerns the social organisation of sleep in various institutional sites and settings. The relationship between dormancy and domicile, as already noted, is a crucial one, but the home is simply one among many places in which sleep occurs. It is not simply a question of organisational rules and regulations, moreover, but of the very architecture of sleep in such settings, so to speak; the places and spaces built for or allocated to sleep, that is to say. Hotels, for example, like private houses, are often spoken of or accounted for in terms of the number of bedrooms, with rooms charged on a per night basis, if not sold in terms of the *quality* of the sleep experience[19]. Boarding schools, in contrast, historically at least, have dormitories, whilst hospitals have wards in which the allocation of 'beds' looms large – part and parcel of the very politics of health care in fact.

So how is sleep organised in such settings and how (well) do its residents or inmates sleep? The following examples, drawn from the broader spectrum of sleeping places and possibilities across the life course, provide instructive comparisons and contrasts.

Pre-school/day-care centres

Children, as noted in Chapter 3, spend a lot of time asleep, in their early years at least. The social organisation of children's sleep in various pre-school sites and settings, in this respect, provides us with a fascinating glimpse of these early ventures across the public–private divide, and of the 'socialisation' processes contained therein.

Day-care, for example, is a prime case in point. This is an area, in the UK at least, where national policies strikingly favour private over public provision. Children's well-being in the pre-school years and their readiness for primary school experience, therefore, 'is stratified' (Mayall 1996: 39; see also Mayall 2002: 144–5). In contrast, for other countries, such as Sweden, Denmark and Japan, pre-school provision, including day-care, is a significant part of children's early lives, whilst their parents are away from home working.

Ben-Ari (1996), for instance, provides us with a fascinating case study of the social organisation of children's nap-time in a Japanese day-care centre. Japan, he notes, comparatively speaking, is an interesting case study, given the 'relative ease of transition' from the intense indulgence and highly charged home context – which includes maternal co-sleeping and co-bathing practices – to the fully demanding and disciplined environment of the school classroom environment (1996: 136). This raises intriguing questions about how this transition is managed or effected given the 'contradictory forces' at work within the home and the pre-school environments. A focus on children's nap-time in such settings, Ben-Ari argues, helps us unravel this apparent contradiction.

In Japan, institutions of early education are differentiated into *yochien* (kindergartens) and *hoikuen* (day-care centres). Kindergartens are usually open half-days, catering to children aged four to five, whilst day-care centres are open all day (often from seven in the morning to six at night). The latter, Ben-Ari (1996: 138) informs us, have shown a great increase over the past few decades, with over 22,000 public or publically available recognised day-care centres catering to over two million children.

As far as sleep in these institutions is concerned, Ben-Ari (1996: 141–2) recounts the following arrangements in one such medium-sized centre, with 22 teachers caring for about 110 children between the ages of three months and six years, mainly from urban middle-class households. Preparation for nap-time begins at around noontime in the hall. The children and teachers clear the hall in which morning activities (such as assembly, games, arts and crafts) have taken place. Next, long mats are rolled out onto the floor. Children and teachers then spread the futons and blankets around the hall. This bedding material is kept in cupboards and taken home once a week for parents to wash ready for the following week. While each child has their own futon, there is no set place where it is put every day. Upon finishing lunch at around 12.30, the children (under the supervision of the teacher) prepare for sleep, which includes going to the toilet, washing hands, brushing teeth and putting on pyjamas. Soft background music is played and the lights are gradually turned off. Then:

> . . . about four or five teachers begin to put children to sleep. Each child is attended by being told 'good night' (oyasumi nasai) and being tucked in. Teachers are careful to wrap the blankets around the children with only their heads protruding. . . . At times teachers softly pat the children on their backs and stomachs in a series of onomatopoeically termed *ton-ton-ton* taps, which very often induce them to sleep. . . . A few minutes before 1:00 the teachers begin to circulate and devote their attention to children who are having trouble falling asleep. Usually they lie

next to these children and softly stroke or caress them. Those trouble-some ones who are *kappatsu* (sprightly) find that the teachers delicately but firmly place their heads below their breasts and their behinds under the adults' knee to calm them. At this stage many teachers actually lie next to the children underneath the latter's blankets with full body con-tact and the exchange of body heat between adults and youngsters. By 1:20 almost all of the children are asleep, and some of the teachers catch a quick nap as well.

(1996: 141)

While the children are asleep the teachers undertake a variety of organisa-tional activities. Then about 2:30 the teachers begin waking the children by gradually turning the lights on. Soft background music again is often played whilst the teachers 'delicately stroke the children, say "good morning" (*ohayo gozaimasu*), and talk with them about their nap' (1996: 142). Some of the teachers again lie down next to the children who have difficulty rous-ing and ease their way back to wakefulness. The whole atmosphere, Ben-Ari (1996: 142) comments, is marked by a 'cozy warmth and tenderness'. After the children have risen, the pre-sleep ritual is carried out in reverse: they visit the toilet; change clothing; arrange their futons; have a light snack; brush teeth, and then start afternoon activities.

Some of these practices may strike the Western observer as strange if not downright problematic or perverse, but in a society where mothers actively and intentionally seek to create ties of dependency with their children, through practices such as co-sleeping and co-bathing, non-verbal commu-nication and indulgence of their desires, some 'carry over' into the pre-school environment is, perhaps, only to be expected. Ben-Ari's prime interest here, however, is with how the Japanese (urban middle class) uti-lize, transfer or add to these strong dyadic and hierarchical ties nurtured at home, wider horizontal ties and orientations to the group. How, in other words, is the '"M" in *mothering* put in parenthesis so that children add *othering* to *(m)othering*?' (1996: 137). What practices such as nap-time imply or reveal, he argues, is the 'inculcation of certain traits and qualities associated with "being Japanese"' (1996: 159). Children's nap-time, in other words, is one form, no more or less, through which day-care centres 'effect the *transfer* of strong relations from the family dyad to the peer group'; a transfer, in effect, of the 'warmth', 'comfortableness', 'commitments' and 'involvement' of children in the dyad at home to the wider group. 'Who sleeps with whom', in this respect, 'continues to be an important question for Japanese throughout their lives' (1996: 159).

As for sleep in schools, rather than pre-schools, suffice to say that pre-cious little occurs, with the exception of that in boarding schools, perhaps, where sleep may or may not take place (see for example Wright 1962 on the school dorm), or the crafty classroom nap behind the teacher's back.

The Japanese art of *inemuri*, yet again, provides an interesting variant on these themes, where napping itself may provide a sign of diligence and commitment to one's studies (Steger 2003a). The home, in short, as these and numerous other examples attest, is clearly not the only place where (pre)school children 'learn' to 'do' sleep. Nor is it the last.

The prison

Two main references spring to mind, to my mind at least, when thinking through the pros and cons of sleep in prisons. The first is Sir Phillip Sydney's famous statement about sleep being the 'prisoner's release', and Shakespeare's notion that 'some must watch while others must sleep'. The second, moving forward in time, concerns Goffman's (1961b) notion of the 'total institution'. Goffman's prime concern here, of course, was the mental hospital or asylum although he recognised that total institutions ranged from monasteries to boarding schools, military barracks, ships or submarines to prisons and the like. A basic social arrangement in modern society, Goffman observes, is that the individual tends to sleep, play and work in different places, with different co-participants, under different authorities, and without an overall rational plan. The central feature of total institutions, in this respect, can be described as:

> . . .a breakdown of the barriers ordinarily separating these three spheres of life. First, all aspects of life are conducted in the same place under the same single authority. Second, each phase of the member's daily activity is carried out in the immediate company of a large batch of others, all of whom are treated alike and required to do the same thing together. Third, all phases of the day's activity are tightly scheduled, with one activity leading at a prearranged time into the next, the whole sequence of activities being imposed from above by a system of explicit formal rulings and a body of officials. Finally, the various enforced activities are brought together into a single rational plan purportedly designed to fulfil the official aims of the institution.
>
> (Goffman 1961b: 17)

We have already glimpsed the nature of prison life in the past through the work of Foucault and others (see Chapter 2 in this book). What, however, of contemporary prison life? How is sleep done 'inside', so to speak?

The first, and perhaps the most obvious point, is that 'doing time', for the prisoner, is itself part and parcel of the punishment. Cohen and Taylor (1972: 86), for example, in their book on the experience of long-term imprisonment, quote Victor Serge (1970) approvingly in this respect. 'Each minute', Serge states, 'may be marvellously – or horribly – profound. . ... There are swift hours and very long seconds. Past time is void. There is no chronology of events to mark it; external duration no longer exists'. Time is also 'marked' in various ways: one can 'tick off certain fixed, definable periods: days, weeks, or months'. This, however, may merely serve to 'bring home the unreality of time even more forcibly' (Cohen and Taylor 1972: 96).

As for the typical prisoner's day, this varies considerably of course from institution to institution. At worst, Fitzgerald and Sim (1979: 51) comment: 'People are locked in their cells all day and night, only getting out to "slop out" and take exercise (weather permitting)'. The usual schedule, however, they inform us, runs something like the following. Up at six o'clock, with the unlocking of cells, following the first count of the day. 'Slopping out', washing, making beds, cleaning cells and breakfast duly follow in the next two hours. Before eight o'clock, those prisoners going to the workshop are counted out of the wing, marched over to the workshop and counted in, with similar counting in/out exercises, including the counting of tools, at lunch-time and at the end of the working day. Exercise is usually taken immediately after lunch, weather permitting. After tea, around about five o'clock, prisoners are usually locked in their cells for a 'quiet hour' which historically 'provided space for personal reflection. It also coincides with the time staff take tea' (1979: 52). In the early evening, prisoners may be unlocked for a recreation period. By about nine o'clock, however:

> . . .prisoners are back in their cells for supper (tea and a bun). Officers begin to lock up, counting as they go from cell to cell. At about ten o'clock the lights go out. Throughout the night, the patrolling officer will look through the peep-hole of each cell to check that the occupants are inside and asleep. For top-security prisoners, the cell light burns all night.
>
> (1979: 51–3)

Overall, Fitzgerald and Sim conclude, echoing the likes of Serge, the most striking feature of daily life in prison is the 'routinized boredom of people passing rather than spending time' (1979: 53).

Perhaps the most recent insights into prison life, albeit from a privileged source, come from (Lord) Jeffery Archer. In volume I of his *Prison Diary*, for example, instructively sub-titled *Hell*, he records a number of sleep-related episodes and incidents. His first destination, Belmarsh Prison in Woolwich, turns out to be a noisy place, which often proves difficult for him. But Archer's first gripe returns us to questions of space and time. Day five of his diary, for instance, informs us that he has been 'incarcerated in a cell five paces by three for twelve and a half hours, and will not be let out again until midday: eighteen and a half hours of solitary confinement. . ... This is Great Britain' (2002: 53). As far as the (night-time) noise of prison life is concerned, the following diary entry on day nine is revealing:

I am awoken in the middle of the night by rap music blasting out from a cell on the other side of the block. . . I'm told that rap music is the biggest single cause of fights breaking out in prison. . . I had to wait until it was turned off before I could get back to sleep. I didn't wake again until eight minutes past six. Amazingly Terry [cell mate] can sleep through anything.

(2002: 98)

Sleep then, returning to Sir Philip Sydney's quote, may well be the prisoner's release, but sleep itself is far from guaranteed for the prisoner doing time.

The hospital: 'dead' tired?

If sleep is a 'great healer', then one may be forgiven for thinking of hospitals as sleep-promoting environments, or at least places where a lot of sleeping takes place. Things, however, are not quite that simple or straightforward. Hospital patients, Martin (2003: 84) declares, are 'routinely subjected to conditions that make normal sleep almost impossible'.

A number of factors may conspire against sound, unencumbered or even unmedicated slumber in hospitals. First and foremost, people may be in acute or chronic, pre- or post-operative, pain or discomfort, which itself of course is a great disrupter of sleep. Tiredness, in turn, makes people more sensitive to pain, thus creating a vicious circle. Second, sleeping in a strange (and possibly uncomfortable) bed, on a ward with other sick and/or snoring if not burping, farting, tossing and turning patients – to say nothing of general hospital noise levels (Souter and Wilson 1986) – may prove disruptive, to say the least. A private room, in this respect, may prove a Godsend. Third, hospital routines themselves and various monitoring exercises, day and night are not exactly planned with sleep in mind, for patients at least. Patients, for example, are routinely woken up very early, further disrupting any sleep they might successfully have gained or snatched throughout the night. One of the worst places imaginable if you need a good night's sleep, according to Martin (2003), is the intensive care unit (ICU). The combination of 'serious illness, serious drugs, constant monitoring, bright lighting and the after-effects of surgery', he argues, 'ensure that the ICU patients are often subjected to severe sleep deprivation': an irony indeed given the fact that the ICU houses 'the sickest people in the hospital, with the greatest need for sleep' (2003: 85).

To these observations, of course, returning to the previous themes of sleep and work, we may add the (chronic) sleep deprivation of hospital staff themselves, including doctors and nurses, who work both day and night to care for the sick.

Viewed in this light, it is probably no exaggeration to say that the hospital is an institutional expression of modern-day sleep deprivation, chronic or otherwise: a place, ironically, where the healing power or therapeutic qualities of sleep are desperately needed yet all too often in short supply. This, I hasten to add, will doubtless vary from patient to patient, ward to ward, if not hospital to hospital, both public and private. As a general statement, nonetheless, it doubtless strikes a chord with many long-suffering (if not 'dead tired') patients and hospital staff alike.

The nursing home

Our final peer into sleep in institutions takes us from one end of the life-course – the pre-school day-care centre – to the other via the nursing home. The nursing home, as Gubrium and Holstein (1999) note, has become a 'paramount site for the care and custody of old people', but it also affects 'how we think about the ageing body'. The classic study here, perhaps, is Townsend's (1962) book *The Last Refuge*. For the best insights into sleeping patterns and practices in such sites and settings, however, we need look no further than Gubrium's (1975) carefully observed study *Living and Dying in Murray Manor*: accounts from a nursing home in the United States.

Sleep, unsurprisingly, turns out to be a crucial part of the picture at *Murray Manor*, including both the sleeping–waking patterns and practices of the residents, clients or patients and the 'bed-body work' of the staff. Sleeping indeed, Gubrium notes, echoing the previous discussion of prison life, is 'another way that patients and residents pass time during the day' (1975: 178) This, in turn, we learn, may occur in 'one's own bed or another's, in lounges, in the lobby, in hallways, in the dining room and at the nurse's station' (1975: 178). Some sleep is 'regularized' and some of it is 'sporadic'. Many residents and patients, for instance, take a nap after lunch. At 'any location on the floors', however, 'seated clientele are likely to doze off if things become monotonous'. Some snore, or drop items they were holding prior to sleep (1975: 178).

When patients sleep in places considered private by others, however, Gubrium notes, a 'commotion' may ensue: caused, on the one hand, through the 'rudeness' of awakening the sleeper, on the other hand, through the 'gall' shown by the intruder in using someone else's private room 'when you have a bed of your own!' (1975: 179). Such is the fracas, indeed, that staff may be called upon to sort it out.

Where one sleeps generally makes a difference to how one's sleep is evaluated by others:

> Sleeping in a bed most of the day is judged negatively but spending nearly as much time sleeping in the Manor's lobby or lounges is considered just a matter of dozing off. The former is believed to be a deliberate plan to *just* sleep, whereas the latter is treated as one of those

things that happens when it gets warm and quiet. Dozing off is defined as an event that 'happens', even though for some patients and residents it happens fairly systematically. At certain times throughout the day, they may be found dozing in specific public places at the Manor.

(1975: 179–80)

In public places, nonetheless, the sleeper is more open to (rude) awakenings, including visitors and the probing or prodding of staff or fellow residents. Sleeping in one's own room or in a private space, in this respect, has its advantages if undisturbed sleep is the goal (1975; 180).

The amount of sleeping that patients and residents do to pass the time did, however, vary considerably in Gubrium's study; some napping for only an hour or so in the afternoon, others retiring to their *made* bed, carefully sleeping *on* them most of the morning and afternoon. There is also, Gubrium observes, a distinct *moral evaluation* of patients and residents in terms of both the *amount* of sleeping they *do,* and the *places* and *spaces* they *do it in*: a point which echoes and amplifies sociological themes first aired in Chapter 3 of this book. Those who sleep their whole days away, for instance, are considered to be just 'whiling all their time away'. *Just* sleeping all day, in other words, may effectively pass the time but it has little or no 'prestige value' for those who do it. Others boast that 'they don't sleep around all day like some others in this place do' (1975: 179): a *normative evaluation* that places them on the right side of the great dividing line between 'doing something' and 'doing nothing' with one's life.

Gubrium provides us with a fascinating series of observations and insights into sleep, not simply in nursing homes, but across the public/private divide in general. We should, however, as previous examples attest, remember the considerable potential for sleep disturbance or disruption that institutional life of any sort can bring, including general noise levels, invasions of privacy and the psychological impact of being there, whether as a patient or a resident (Morgan 1987). Sleeping tablets or pills, moreover, alongside other medications, are another important part of the story in managing or regulating sleeping/waking life in institutional sites and settings of this kind.

There is, however, a further more troubling or sinister dimension to these issues, which is not so much about sleep, per se, but about the 'hidden work' of the nursing home in terms of 'bedroom abuse'. Much bed-and-body work, to be sure, goes on in the nursing home behind the scenes, so to speak, including caring and cleaning, washing and dressing; duties which are all too often physically hard and dirty. This hidden bedroom work, as Lee-Treweek's (2001) 'Cedar Court' nursing home study reveals, is often undertaken by low status workers whose 'product' is then presented to, and by, higher status workers: a primal Goffmanesque drama of front-stage, back-stage work, in effect, in which the sanitized person is then put on display for visitors in the lounge. Depersonalisation and mistreatment may arise in such contexts, Lee-Treweek (2001: 235) suggests, as another facet of this bedroom-based work. Punishment and mistreatment, for instance, may help 'create the "lounge standard patient" which, paradoxically, indicates that care is "being carried out"'. Within this hidden bedroom world, moreover, non-physical abuse is 'very difficult for trained staff, visitors or others to perceive': a 'hard' yet 'invisible' culture, in effect, which takes place behind closed doors (2001: 235).

From dozing in the lounge to bed-and-body work, the nursing home reveals much about the public and private world of sleeping and waking life, including the hidden dimensions or underside of social organisations and institutions, both past and present, in which much front-stage, back-stage, work goes on, good or bad.

Homelessness: nowhere to sleep?

The flip side of these arguments and insights into sleeping in social organisations and institutions, concerns the problem of having 'nowhere to sleep', or 'sleeping rough' to be more precise – everybody sleeps somewhere, of course, whether the place is desirable or otherwise.

George Orwell's (2003/1933) vivid memoir of his time amongst the poor and destitute in London and Paris, for instance, is a veritable treasure trove of insights into the sleeping and waking lives of the 'down and out'; a painstaking documentation of a world of unrelenting drudgery and squalor, living among tramps, surviving on scraps and cigarette butts, working as a dishwasher in the vile 'Hotel X' and sleeping in bug-infested hostels and doss houses. Work as a *plongeur* in the hotel, for example, taught Orwell: 'the true value of sleep, just as being hungry had taught me the true value of food. Sleep had ceased to be a mere physical necessity. It was something voluptuous, a debauch more than a relief' (2003/1933: 96). As for the joys of the London doss house and the need for a 'good kip', Orwell informs us that the bed was as:

> . . . hard as a board, and as for the pillow, it was a mere hard cylinder like a block of wood, it was worse than sleeping on a table. . . . The sheets stank so horribly of sweat that I could not bear them near my nose. . . .. Several noises recurred throughout the night. About once an hour the man on my left. . . woke up, swore vilely and lighted a cigarette. Another man, victim of bladder disease, got up and noisily used his chamber pot half a dozen times during the night. The man in the corner had a coughing fit once every twenty minutes. . . . Every time he coughed or the other man swore, a sleepy voice from one of the beds cried out 'shut up, oh, for Christ's sake, shut up!' I had about an hour's sleep in all.
>
> (2003/1933: 139)

The problems of homelessness, of course, have not gone away since Orwell's time: if only they had. Various estimates, for example, suggest that there could be as many as 100,000 single homeless people in London alone. Homeless people, moreover, have diverse experiences, circumstances, prospects and hopes; for some homelessness is a temporary problem, for others it is a recurring problem (see, for example, www.homelesspages.org.uk; www.shelter.org.uk; and the British Government's recent strategy document on rough sleeping, *Coming in From the Cold* [Office of the Deputy Prime Minister, 1999]).

It is not simply a case of rough sleeping being tough, however, but of various authorities and (corporate) interests getting tough on rough sleeping. In Los Angeles, for example, a place of great contrasts between wealth and poverty, efforts have been made to eliminate vagrancy as property developers spot the potential for profitable housing blocks for employees of e-commerce companies and the entertainment industry. A zero-tolerance policy on the part of the LA Police Department regarding street-sleepers has emerged in this context, as pressure on City Hall to revive the city centre intensifies (Campbell 2000).

Rensen's (2003) recent ethnographic work on sleeping rough in Amsterdam casts further light on these issues. Taking as his point of departure Spradley's (1970) claim that sleep is an 'act embodying numerous facets of homelessness' and Dunier's (2000) attempts to understand sleeping on the sidewalks within the 'overall logic' of homeless people's lives, Rensen seeks to answer the question of 'why' the rough sleepers or 'urban nomads' of Amsterdam sleep outside? In doing so, he points to three main factors that operate at the micro, meso and macro levels respectively: first, the influence of personal attributes such as addiction or mental illness; second, the opportunities for autonomy that the urban environment offers homeless individuals; third, rules established in the care organisations for the homeless in Amsterdam (2003: 88). Sleep, Rensen shows, is a 'rare privilege' for the majority of outside sleepers. Even resting is 'scarcely possible'. The homeless, in this sense, may exist in a liminal state somewhere between fatigue and 'half sleep'. Bad weather conditions, police control, the lack of security, the cycle of day and night, are obvious factors here in accounting for this liminal state of affairs. The 'magnetic appeal of the street', the rules of social care and personal attributes such as drug addiction, however, are equally important influences. 'Half sleep', in this respect, is a response to these exigencies and the prime way, in Rensen's opinion, that rough sleepers try to fight exhaustion (2003: 101).

Sleeping outside, as this suggests, is almost always a 'compromise'. In general nevertheless, Rensen maintains, rough sleepers remain 'ambivalent' about the meaning of sleep and rest:

Rest, at a given time, is both important and unimportant. Because it is so difficult to obtain, sleep is a central theme in their lives. To prevent exhaustion they have to take their chance in order to get rest. *They often wonder where and when they will get sleep.* But other aspects of their lives, such as earning money, are also important. Because of that, sleep becomes something *to take as it comes, to postpone.* A lot of rough sleepers are *exhausted at times* but they try not to think about it. *The logic of homelessness thus implies a certain degree of indifference towards rest.*

(2003: 105, my emphasis)

This gives rise to another important distinction, namely that the homeless who sleep inside social care institutions are more similar to the non-homeless (whose sleeping place is more or less taken-for-granted), than to rough sleepers; a fact, Rensen (2003: 106) concludes, that is underestimated in the literature on 'homelessness' to date.

To this, of course, returning to the likes of Goffman (1981/1963), we may add the stigmatising costs or consequences of rough sleeping, *qua* 'deviant' sleep role, whether *felt* or *enacted*[20]. There is perhaps a final irony here, however: whilst Rensen is right to refer to the *embedment* of sleep in the lives of these rough-sleepers – part and parcel of the overall 'logic' of their lives, that is to say – they are also quite literally *dis-embedded* as well as dis-empowered when it comes to sleep, if by that one means without proper bed or abode. Sleep, in short, may well be embedded in all our lives, but it is only the favoured or fortunate among us whose embodiment is truly embedded whilst we sleep, night or day.

Sleep, torture and human rights

These considerations of sleeping rough or sleep and homelessness are also part and parcel of a broader set of questions and issues concerning sleep and human rights. Already, casting our minds back to Chapter 3, we have viewed sleep not simply as a *resource* but as a basic human *right*: one that casts further important light on the gender division of labour and the (dis)advantage contained therein. The 'politics of sleep', that is to say.

Another interesting example or illustration of these principles in practice occurred through a landmark ruling by the European Court of Human Rights, which upheld the right of Heathrow airport residents to a sound night's sleep: a ruling with important implications for millions of people troubled by aircraft noise (Brown 2001; *Hatton and others v. the UK*, European Court of Human Rights, 2 October 2001).

Each of the eight residents, who had been battling for ten years against night flights, was awarded £4,000 damages for loss of sleep, plus a total of £70,000 to pay legal costs and expenses (Brown 2001). The Court accepted the residents' basic premise that it was a human right to have a good night's sleep and invited the Department of Transport to make a case for depriving them of it. The Court ruled five to two that the government had breached Article 8 of the European Convention of Human Rights, because the 'State failed to strike a fair balance between the UK's economic well-being and the applicant's effective enjoyment of their right to respect for their homes and their private family lives'. The eight successful residents represented thousands of people who had petitioned the government over night flights and had twice won judicial reviews against the government without getting flights stopped (Brown 2001).

Loss of this basic human right, however, may stem from other more troubling or sinister sources. A violent or abusive domestic relationship, for example, may leave its mark in many ways, including sleep problems. These problems, moreover, may well persist long after the violence or abuse has ended. As most domestic abuse is against women this provides yet another dimension to gender inequalities. Hathaway and colleagues' (2000) population-based health survey, for example, found that 53% of women reporting partner violence had experienced problems getting enough sleep compared to 28% of women not reporting violence. Brokaw and colleagues (2002) also found that nightmares were a common problem. In a recent study of general practitioners, moreover, doctors stated that abused women often initially attended the surgery complaining of sleeping problems (Taft et al 2004). Women's own disturbed sleep may, in turn, impact on their children. Studies have documented sleep disturbance in children whilst they are living in a household where their mothers are subjected to abuse (Lemmey et al 2001), but also found that sleep problems may continue after they have resettled (Mertin and Mohr 2002).

Our own pilot work with women in refuges following domestic violence, confirms this picture (Williams, Humphreys and Lowe 2004). Key themes in the focus groups with these women included the following: being woken or stopped from sleeping as part of the abuse ('don't you dare go to sleep'); being afraid to sleep too deeply; fear of being attacked or even killed whilst asleep; taking/timing sleep when perpetrators were out or asleep themselves; fighting constant fatigue and other physical signs of sleep deprivation (headaches, body aches); use of alcohol, street or prescription drugs to manage sleep; and, continuing 'bad' sleep (including bad dreams) after the domestic violence had ended, particularly when court cases or child contact was imminent. The impact of domestic violence on children's sleep was also a prominent theme in these women's accounts. Women, in this respect, often talked of feeling that they had 'let the children down' and of 'not liking to fall asleep before your kids', given their children's own vulnerabilities and sleep problems, including disturbed sleep, reluctance to go to sleep, night waking, bed-wetting, and episodes of shouting or crying in their sleep. Consequently, even when re-housed, children were often put to bed together for reassurance: a sort of safety in numbers approach.

Another human rights issue is the sad and sorry tale of deliberate attempts, around the world, to deprive people of sleep in the name of interrogation, punishment or torture. Sleep deprivation of this kind has a long history. Martin (2003) comments, that it may have served as a form of capital punishment in China in the not so dim and distant past, for example. King Perseus of Macedonia, de Montaigne informs us, when a prisoner in Rome, was *'done to death* by being prevented from sleeping' (1991/1572, my emphasis). Sleep deprivation, moreover, has been used to 'soften up' prisoners and make them talk for centuries. Communists in the Korean War of 1950–53, for instance, tortured Americans and Allied Prisoners of War by systematically depriving them of sleep. In this confused, fatigued and fearful state, they were ready and willing to confess to (m)any crimes, real or imaginary, or even 'cross-sides' and condemn the USA (Martin 2003: 72). The UK is also no stranger to such tactics. Thirty years ago, for example, British security forces in Belfast decided to use five main interrogation techniques against IRA suspects. These techniques, which had been finessed by the KGB, were hooding, noise bombardment, food and water deprivation, sleep deprivation and being forced to stand for long periods spread-eagled against the wall (www.torturecare.org.uk).

One of the most recent, well publicised, manifestations of these principles in practice, concerns the treatment meted out by US military personnel to some of the Abu Ghraib prisoners in Iraq. These methods included stress and duress techniques such as sleep deprivation, noise bombardment, and forcing prisoners to stand in contorted positions for prolonged periods of time, to say nothing of other alleged abuses such as punching, slapping, kicking, threats of execution, 'water boarding', the use of dogs to terrorize, the wearing of hoods, and various unsavoury sexual acts. These so-called 'stress and duress' techniques, moreover, have been widely alleged by former detainees held in US custody in Afghanistan, some of whom were subsequently transferred to Guantánamo Bay. Secretary of State Rumsfeld assured a Senate Committee that Pentagon lawyers had approved these (euphemistically described) 'sleep management', 'dietary manipulation' and 'stress position' techniques, which were 'deemed to be consistent with the Geneva Conventions'. According to Amnesty International, however, 'these techniques of torture or cruel, inhuman, degrading treatments, are grave breaches of the Fourth Geneva Convention, amounting to war crimes, and violate the Convention Against Torture, to which the USA is a state party' (Amnesty International 2005).

To these observations concerning tactics or techniques of 'sleep management', 'manipulation' or 'deprivation', we may add other ways in which the horrors of war impact either directly or indirectly on people's sleep. Prolonged sleep deprivation, for instance, was the cause of many of the psychiatric casualties of World War I (Martin 2003). Continuous shelling, it seems, broke men for reasons other than simply shell shock; it deprived them of sleep. Doctors, Martin (2003: 73) notes, often found that when a man with disabling shell shock was granted respite from the front line, he would 'rapidly recover and be able to return to his unit within days'. 'Getting a few nights' sleep within the hospital', in other words, 'probably did more good than the psychotherapy that went with it' (2003: 73) (see also the earlier section of this chapter on sleep and the military).

Primo Levi's (1987/1958) moving account of life in a concentration camp (Auschwitz), provides another telling testimony of the trials and tribulations of sleep under extreme, inhumane conditions (see also Alexander Solzhenitsyn's 1968, *One Day in the Life of Ivan Denisovich*). Sleep, in this respect, may prove precious but elusive, particularly with a troublesome bed-mate in a bed with a width little more than two feet:

> Back against back, I struggle to regain a reasonable area of the straw mattress; with the base of my back I exercise a progressive pressure against his back; then I turn around and try to push with my knees. . ... But it is all in vain: he is much heavier than me and seems to turn to stone in his sleep. . ... So I adapt myself to lie like this, forced into immobility, half lying on the wooden edge. Nevertheless I am so tired and stunned that I, too, soon fall asleep and seem to be sleeping on the tracks of a rail road. . .*I have my eyes closed and I do not want to open them lest my sleep escape me.*
>
> (Levi 1987/1958: 65)

Sleep then, as these diverse references suggest, is not simply a personal but a political, legal and ethical issue; a basic human *right*, whether honoured or breached, respected or abused. Placing these issues in a global perspective, moreover, provides an important reminder of the fitful or fateful, fragile or fragmented sleep of those who, through poverty, famine, war and the like, live their lives 'on the edge', both literally and metaphorically. Sleep deprivation, in this respect, harking back to previous comments in this chapter, comes in many shapes and sizes around the world, some more troubling and disturbing than others.

Conclusions

A number of conclusions may be drawn from this chapter concerning the social patterning and social organisation of sleep.

First, debates as to whether or not society is (chronically) sleep deprived are not only far from settled, but part and parcel of broader issues to do with social, economic and technological transformation in general, and the changing *pace* or *tempo* of life and living in particular. Sleep, in this respect, lies at the nexus of debates on 'speeding up' and 'slowing down' in late or postmodernity, co-opted, in different ways, to both causes. The sleep 'crisis', as this suggests, is a knotty issue to disentangle. On the one hand, (chronic) sleep deprivation may very well be a 'real' problem for many people today in our 24/7 society. On the other hand, we should also recognise or entertain the possibility that *part of the problem* here (if problem it is) concerns a (new) readiness and willingness, within professional and popular if not lay culture, to frame or translate all manner of problems and issues into sleep-related matters; a process which itself engenders a sleep 'crisis' of sorts that is more apparent than real given the cipher-like quality of sleep. There may, moreover, be differential class propensities to do so, which itself may go some way towards explaining recent findings of a greater self-assessed sleep deficit amongst managers and other white-collar workers. Elements of *both* these explanations in all likelihood are correct, and much more besides, thereby obviating the need to take sides in these debates. What is clear, nonetheless, for better or worse, is that the politics of sleep in the 24/7 era are now moving 'out of the bedroom, home and neighbourhood, and into the courts, boardroom and even parliament' (Crossley 2004: 28).

Second, the notion of cultures of sleep alerts us to important international, intercultural and historical variations in sleeping patterns and practices around the world, both past and present, including *monophasic*, *biphasic* (or *siesta*) and *polyphasic* sleep cultures. The polyphasic pattern it seems is becoming increasingly popular, and may prove to be the future pattern of choice in the global age, as the *flexible*, *efficient* or *smart* way to sleep. Any such emergent trends, however, are likely to be contingent, if not contradictory, depending, amongst other things, on socio-economic factors and the socio-cultural context of change.

Third, following directly on from these previous two points, work, it is clear, has important implications for our sleep as well as our waking lives, both positive and negative. How important this is of course depends on many factors, including personal characteristics or predispositions, the nature and type of work we do and the broader social and economic climate and context within which it occurs. The relationship between work time, work culture, work ethics and sleep, as this suggests, is a complex one, with or without any mention of the modern-day work stress phenomenon or 'epidemic'; itself the subject of much controversy and debate. Historical comparison with previous generations of workers, moreover, yields a mixed bag of 'gains' and 'losses' as far as the modern-day worker is concerned. What is evident, nonetheless, is that a growing discourse and debate in late/postmodernity surrounds the risks of sleepiness at work, personified in figures as diverse as the drowsy lorry driver and the sleepy (junior) hospital doctor. Whether or not this construction of 'sleepy workers' promotes the identity of 'passive victim' found in the work stress discourse – one that is 'agency-robbing' and conservative in its implications – is a moot point. There are nonetheless instructive parallels or similarities here between some of the (therapeutic) assumptions embedded within the work stress discourse and some of the claim-making surrounding sleepy workers.

The (not so) humble nap also tells us much about the changing fate or fortunes of sleep, both inside and outside the workplace; an uneven or variable trend in terms of the mental–manual division of labour which itself may simply superimpose new inequalities on old ones. The jury is still very much out on the merits of the workplace nap *qua* flexible friend or foe. The military, meanwhile, have gone one or more steps further down the line here, combating sleep on a number of fronts, including wakefulness-promoting drugs and other forms of technological trickery: a sign of things to come perhaps on or off the battlefield.

The social patterning/organisation of sleep in various institutions adds further important insights and dimensions to these debates, including sleep(lessness) in day-care centres, prisons, hospitals and nursing homes; places, as we have seen, which take us from infancy to old age. The relationship between dormancy and domicile, moreover, is thrown into critical relief in the case of 'rough' sleepers. Herein lies the fifth conclusion then concerning not simply the *siting* or *situating* of sleep(lessness) but the (dis)embedment of sleep in peoples lives and the (dis)advantages it conceals and reveals.

The final, and perhaps most important conclusion, however, concerns the fact that sleep, whether honoured or breached, is a basic human *right* as well as a *resource*. From gender inequalities in the domestic milieu, through the struggle of residents to ban night-time flights, to domestic violence, torture, interrogation techniques and the horrors of war, the lines of these injustices and the deprivations they engender can be traced. To deprive someone of sleep, in this respect, may or may not be legitimate, depending on the circumstances and the context in question, but sooner or later it leads, or should lead, to a court of appeal where this basic human right is vindicated rather than violated. Placing these issues in a global perspective, moreover, reminds us of the perilous or precarious sleep of many people around the world, both past and present, due to atrocities and disasters of various kinds. Sleep, in this respect, is a universal human imperative that, at one and the same time, unites and divides us: a shared vulnerability that is open to all manner of 'rights' and 'wrongs'. The politics of sleep indeed!

Notes

1 I do not, in what follows, wish to take sides in these debates. The debate, instead, and the claim-making surrounding it is what is most important, sociologically speaking, for the purposes of this chapter: the social framing or production of a 'problem', that is to say, in which drowsiness or (excessive) daytime sleepiness

looms large. See also Kroll-Smith (2000) on the social production of the 'drowsy person' and Chapter 5 in this book, for its therapeutic ramifications.

2 Measures of sleepiness range from those taken in the sleep laboratory, such as the Stanford developed Multiple Sleep Latency Test (Carskadon et al 1982) – a measure that records the time taken for an individual connected to an EEG machine to fall asleep whilst lying on a comfortable bed in a darkened room; the longer the sleep latency the less sleepy the subject – to self-administered, widely used instruments such as the Epworth Sleepiness scale (Johns 1991). See Morgan (1987: Ch. 1) for a useful discussion of the history of sleep and sleepiness measurement, and Partinen and Hublin (2000) on some of the methodological difficulties of epidemiological studies of (excessive) daytime sleepiness. To test your own sleepiness score using the Epworth Sleepiness Scale, go to www.sleepfoundation.org/epworth/quiz.cfm.

3 As far as sleep *quality* goes, however, the majority of American adults (73%) rate it as 'good', 'very good' or 'excellent', while 40% rate their sleep quality as 'excellent' or 'very good' (NSF 2003).

4 The 'overwhelmingly dominant predictor' of sleeping habits, in Blaxter's (1990) study, was health status, which in turn led her to conclude, rightly or wrongly, 'that the use of sleeping habits as another "voluntary" behaviour (in a survey at one moment of time) does not appear justified' (1990: 127).

5 The UK 2000 Time Use Survey, for example, paints a somewhat different picture, with eight-year-olds sleeping on average nearly 11 hours a night, reducing to under 10 hours per night by the age of 13. By the time people reach their mid-20s sleep time is less than nine hours but then sleep remains fairly constant at around eight hours until people get into their 60s and beyond, when it begins to rise towards a nine hour average. Females, on the whole, appear to sleep longer than males, particularly in the 30–60 age range (ONS 2003).

6 The Demos study – a MORI poll of a representative sample of 1,006 British adults interviewed by telephone in June 2004 – found that self-assessed sleep 'deficit' or 'deprivation' was most concentrated amongst the people in the 25–54 age bracket (i.e. those of working age who are likely to have family responsibilities), managers and white-collar workers (51%) and full-time workers (49%). Women, interestingly, were only 'marginally' more likely than men to say they did not get enough sleep: 40% of women compared to 37% of men. The sleep 'deficit' appeared to be geographically concentrated in London and the South East, due perhaps to factors such as commuting times, long work hours and environmental noise. As for the consequences of sleep deprivation, people reported a greater likelihood of irritability and shouting, mistakes at work and behind the wheel of a car, and of falling asleep at work. Key factors identified as disruptors of sleep were children (41% of parents reported their sleep was disrupted by children waking), worry at work (15% of managers say they worry about work), and noise from the street, traffic, animals and neighbours (Leadbeater 2004).

7 Thanks to Charles Leadbeater for discussion of these issues, both in general and in relation to his own Demos report.

8 There have, in fact, been recent cases where the wrecklessly sleepy have been prosecuted. The Selby rail disaster in Britain, for example, is a case in which a dozing driver caused ten deaths when his vehicle slid from the road onto a railway line resulting in the subsequent rail crash. The judge concluded that driving whilst sleepy was as bad as drunk-driving, and the sentenced defendant – whom he dismissed as 'arrogant' in believing he could make a 150-mile journey after staying up all night on the telephone to a woman friend – to five years imprisonment (Wainwright 2002).

9 It may, of course, Li acknowledges, be an exaggeration to claim that sleep patterns are indicators of the level of socio-economic development of a country, but 'undoubtedly', he claims, 'the position where society stands on the ladder of economic growth or modernization underlies the diverging attitudes towards these patterns' (2003: 62).

10 Benedict (1989/1946), for example, in *The Chrysanthemum and the Sword*, refers to sleep being ruthlessly sacrificed for 'serious affairs' in Japanese culture. She also notes how, compared to the American emphasis on sleep for energy and efficiency, the Japanese sleep for other reasons and gladly go to sleep when 'the coast is clear'.

11 This is not to deny the importance of other types of unpaid 'work', of course, such as voluntary work, home workers and carers. It is paid work, however, for the purposes of this particular chapter that provides the main focus of inquiry given the discourse and debate that surrounds it. See also Chapter 3 in this book, for a discussion of sleep in relation to the gendered division of labour at home.

12 In Doi and Minowa's (2003) study of gender difference in excessive daytime sleepiness (EDS) amongst Japanese workers – full-time, non-manual, non-shift employees working at a telecommunications company in the Tokyo metropolitan area – the prevalence rates for EDS were 13.3% for women and 7.2% for men. A ban on overtime and the provision of 'mental health hygiene', these authors conclude, are important *general strategies* for reducing EDS at worksites. In the case of women, the formation of effective strategies for improving women's status at home and in the workplace (promoting gender equality in the division of labour at home, for example, and strengthening family care policies for working women) must also be a solution to the prevention of EDS.

13 A European World Health Organization 'working group' (WHO 2004), for example, produced a complex model of the impact of various stimuli and stressors on sleep and health status. This included: (i) biological and psychological predispositions; (ii) external stimuli such as noise, temperature, light and 'psychosocial demand'; (iii) 'evening mind state'; (iv) sleep indicators such as fragmentation, arousals, reduction, awakening and satisfaction with sleep quality; and (v) health and social consequences, such as self medication, sleepiness, accidents, fatigue, depression, obesity, cardiovascular disease, hypertension and diabetes. Only some of these links, the working group notes, have been 'proven', with complex feedback loops included within the model.

14 A total of 58% of union health and safety representatives, according to the TUC (2002) survey, cite stress as the major cause of complaints – outstripping conditions such as back pain and repetitive strain injury. Public sector workers were more likely to complain of stress than those in the private sector. Although being overloaded with work was the commonest cause, there was a slight rise in complaints of stress due to redundancies (Hinsliff 2004).

15 Thanks to Charles Leadbeater for discussion of these issues.

16 There is in fact, technically speaking, something known as 'sleep efficiency' – the percentage of time between falling asleep and waking up that you actually spend asleep – which in turn provides a measure of sleep *quality*: how continuous or uninterrupted your sleep has been, that is to say (Martin 2003: 109). My use of the term here, however, denotes the broader associations between sleep and efficiency today, in the workplace and beyond, which include but extend far beyond these technical measures and meanings.

17 It is not so much a case of napping *on* the job, as Anthony and Anthony are at pains to point out, but of napping *at* the job: a difference, they argue, that can 'make or break an organization's attitudes towards workplace napping' (2001:

13). The next major napping 'breakthrough' will come, they claim, 'when employers recognize that people can nap *and* work at the same time': a case of 'napping *while* working' (2001: 23).

18 As I write, in fact, the story has just broken in the British press that 'The Ministry of Defence (MoD) bought thousands of stay-awake pills in advance of war in Iraq' (Sample and Evans 2004).

19 Mention should also be made here of the latest Japanese import: the short-stay capsule hotel which is claimed to pack a lot of luxury into a little space. Simon Woodroffe, the man behind the Yo! Sushi chain of restaurants, has brought the concept from Japan and plans to build the 'Yotels' throughout Britain. For £10 per hour or £75 per night, guests will be able to sleep in rooms measuring 10 square metres and without any proper windows. All pods, nonetheless, will have flat screen TVs, a rotating bed to save space and will be connected up to broadband, with the lighting designed 'aeroplane style'. These space-saving hotels, it is reported, have been hugely popular in Japan, where they are often located near railway stations, catering to business people or commuters who want a bit of shut-eye or have missed the last train home. One in central Tokyo, for example, has more than 600 pods (Scott 2004: 5).

20 Felt stigma refers to the subjective feelings of embarrassment or shame attached to a particular status or condition, whereas enacted stigma refers to actual episodes of stigmatisation by others; see Scambler (1989).

Chapter 5

Colonising/capitalising on sleep? Medicalisation and beyond . . .

Introduction

In this final chapter we take a further look at the fate of sleep in the current era, with particular reference to debates concerning the medicalisation/ healthicisation of sleep and the 'colonisation' of sleep through a variety of 'dormant expertise'. In doing so we also consider, toward the end of the chapter, the intersections between these trends and developments and other, more general, processes of commercialisation/commodification surrounding sleep in late or postmodernity. This, in turn, provides the basis for some further sociological reflections, in a more speculative vein, on what, for want of a better phrase, might be termed the 'sleepicisation' of society.

It is to the first of these issues, therefore, that we now turn, revisiting, revising and updating the medicalisation thesis in the process.

The medicalisation thesis revisited

Debates concerning the medicalisation of society have raged over the years, on a number of fronts and from a variety of quarters. The lines of these debates can be traced from Zola's (1972) deliberations on the medicalisation of life to Freidson's (1970) notion of medicine as a moral enterprise, and from Illich's (1975) critique of iatrogenic medicine to feminist debates on the medicalisation of women's bodies and reproductive lives (Oakley 1984, Martin 1987). To this we may add the detection of supposed counter-trends concerning the 'demedicalisation' of society (Fox 1977), debates as to the 'gains' as well as the 'losses' associated with medicalisation (Reisman 1989), together with the raising of important questions surrounding imperialist motive and intent on the part of sociology and medicine alike (Strong 1979, Conrad and Schneider 1980, Williams 2001). Orthodox medicalisation critiques, moreover, have themselves been eclipsed in recent years by other more thoroughgoing Foucauldian critiques in which the very notion of demedicalisation, or a return to the 'authentic' body, is further problematised (Lupton 1997). There has also been growing recognition of what Conrad (2004), commenting on trends and developments in the US, has recently termed the 'shifting engines of medicalization', including biotechnology (particularly the pharmaceutical industry and genetics), consumers and managed care markets (see also Conrad and Leiter 2004; Clarke et al 2003)[1].

At least four important issues, for our purposes, emerge from these debates. First and foremost, medicalisation is a complex, multifaceted process that consists of 'defining a problem in medical terms, using medical language to describe the problem, adopting a medical framework to under-stand a problem, or using a medical intervention to "treat" it' (Conrad 1992: 211). Medicalisation may occur on a number of different levels, including the *interactional* level (e.g. face-to-face doctor–patient relations), the *conceptual* level (e.g. when a medical vocabulary is used to describe a 'problem'), and the *institutional* level (e.g. when organisations use a medical approach to manage or control a particular problem) (Conrad and Schneider 1980). Rarely if ever, then, can medicalisation be cast in simple yes/no, either/or terms. Thinking about *levels* and *degrees* of medicalisation in relation to particular problems and issues over time, in this respect, is the best way forward in most cases. Second, we should be alive to the different drivers of these processes over time, including the role of the media and the Internet, as well as the factors mentioned above. Third, questions of *imperialist* motive or intent cannot be equated or conflated with the medicalisation process per se, nor should imperialism provide an evaluative criteria in assessing the validity of such critiques. The value of the medicalisation thesis, in contrast, lies in the processes it seeks to explain, not the sociological motives underpinning it or the intentions of the medical profession (Conrad and Schneider 1980). Medicalisation, as this suggests, is a socio-cultural process that '*may or may not* involve the medical profession, lead to med-ical social control or treatment, or be the result of *intentional expansion by the medical profession*' (Conrad 1992: 211, my emphasis). Fourth, a dis-tinction may usefully be drawn here, in Conrad's (1992) terms, between medicalisation and 'healthicisation': the former advancing biomedical causes and interventions, the latter advancing lifestyle explanations and behavioural interventions. The two of course, in reality, are closely interre-lated, given the rise of what Armstrong (1995) terms 'surveillance medicine' crystallised in a web of lifestyle risk factors. Medicalisation however, Conrad argues, turns the moral into the medical, whilst healthicisation turns health into the moral (1992: 223). As for questions surrounding the medicalisation or demedicalisation of society (the above Foucauldian cri-tiques notwithstanding), whilst the weight of evidence continues to point towards processes of medicalisation, this, Conrad stresses, must be seen as a 'bi-directional process' (1992: 226).

Recent studies in this vein have focused on issues as diverse as chronic fatigue syndrome (CFS) (Broom and Woodward 1996), repetitive strain injury (RSI) (Arksey 1998), and even Gulf war syndrome (Showalter 1997, Bury 1997). But what about sleep?

The medicalisation of sleep?

> *Sleep is that golden chain that ties health and our bodies together* (Thomas Dekker, *The Guls Horne-Booke*, 1969/1609)

> *Dochtúir na sláinte an codladh [Health's doctor is sleep]* (old Gaelic saying)

Is sleep yet *another* or even the *latest* chapter in the medicalisation story? To ask this question, of course, begs further or prior historical questions as to what exactly 'latest' means and when precisely any such trends began. There are, to be sure, important historical precursors one might point to here, particularly in the nineteenth century, as Chapter 2 in this book attests. Let me, however, in this chapter, focus primarily on recent trends and current developments, set against the backdrop of these previous historical themes and issues, if not 'premonitions' of things to come. What, in other words, is the current situation as far as the medicalisation of sleep is concerned, and what recent trends and developments explain this state of affairs, good, bad or indifferent? The answer, unsurprisingly perhaps in the light of the foregoing points and issues, is far from simple or straightforward.

Certainly, there is plenty of evidence of (chronic) sleep deprivation in our midst, as we saw in Chapter 4; another important dimension, it seems, of today's risk society (Beck 1992, Giddens 1991). But the (chronic) sleep deprivation thesis, as we also saw, is open to dispute on a number of counts. Evidence for the (chronic) sleep deprivation thesis, including claims as to its costs and consequences, at best provides only limited support for the medicalisation thesis. Sleep deprivation, for example, is clearly not synonymous with sleep pathology or sleep disorders, in the medical sense of the word, and sleepiness may be seen, rightly or wrongly, as a 'normal' part of everyday life. We need to dig more deeply into these issues and to look elsewhere for answers to these questions.

It is tempting, on further inspection, to conclude that the medicalisation of sleep has not occurred to any significant degree to date. Much criticism, for example, has been leveled at the lack of attention to sleep matters, let alone sleep disorders, in medicine today, including claims that both medical and lay 'ignorance' is the worst sleep disorder of all (Dement with Vaughan 2000). People's reluctance to take sleep troubles to their doctors, or even to recognize that they may have a sleep problem if not an underlying disorder, is matched or mirrored by doctors' own neglect or reluctance to inquire or intervene in sleep-related matters in routine, front-line, day-to-day clinical practice. Approximately 40 million people in the United States, according to the National Commission on Sleep Disorders Research (1993), suffer from a chronic sleep disorder, and an additional 20–30 million are affected by intermittent sleep-related problems of one form or another. An overwhelming majority of these problems nevertheless, it is claimed, remain 'undiagnosed and untreated'. In a National Sleep Foundation primary care physician survey (NSF 2000), for instance, nearly half (48%) of doctors surveyed 'rarely', 'occasionally', or 'never', screened their patients for sleep problems.

This in turn is linked to a lack of medical training in sleep matters. Only a quarter (25%) of doctors in the aforementioned NSF survey (2000), for example, had had six or more hours of courses in sleep medicine. The same, it seems, goes for UK doctors (in training): a recent study, for instance, found that the median total time devoted to sleep and its disorders in UK undergraduate medical teaching was five minutes. For pre-clinical teaching this rose to 15 minutes, with a flat zero recorded for clinical teaching (Stores and Crawford 1998). As in other countries, these authors conclude that 'undergraduate medical teaching is inadequate as a basis for the development of competence in diagnosing and treating sleep disorders, which are common and cause difficulties in all sections of the population' (Stores and Crawford 1998: 149; see also Currie et al. 2005). This, coupled with the fact that many sleep specialists are not in fact medically trained or qualified, underlines the contention or conviction that sleep is not in fact a very medicalised phenomenon, to date at least: an apparent disjunction, that is to say, between the supposed 'epidemic' of problems, if not sleep disorders, in our midst today, and a lack of clinical attention to these matters to date.

On the other hand, of course, many millions of prescription hypnotics are still dished out each year by doctors to their tired and weary patients, particularly to women and the elderly, despite various scares and controversies over the years. In England, for example, the total volume of general practitioner prescriptions for hypnotics showed a 'modest decline' from 13.6 million in 1980 to 10.6 million in 2000 (a fall of 22%). During the same period, prescriptions for anxiolytics fell from 18.9 million to 5.9 million (a 69% fall) (Morgan et al 2004; see also the *Drugs and Therepeutics Bulletin* 2004)[2]. Similar trends have been reported elsewhere in Europe. As a result of these differential trajectories, 'most prescriptions for benzodiazepines have been for hypnotic rather than anxiolytic products', which in turn clearly indicates a 'robust demand for insomnia management amongst NHS clinicians' and a 'clear need to recognize the role of insomnia management in benzodiazepine reduction' (Morgan et al. 2004: 1). Indeed, sleeping tablets or pills are one of the most commonly prescribed drugs at the primary health care level (Partinen and Hublin 2000). Women and the elderly, to repeat, may be particularly vulnerable to the medicalisation of their sleep 'problems' in this way (Gabe and Bury 1996a; Hislop and Arber 2003c), despite effective alternative forms of treatment (Holdbrook 2004; Morgan 1987; Morgan et al 2004; see also Gabe 2001 and Gabe and Bury 1996b on the Halcion controversy/crisis).

As for the apparent disjunction between sleep problems and clinical concerns, this itself has provided the basis for a growing number of rallying calls, in recent years, from various quarters, for doctors and the public alike to wake up to the importance of sleep in general and the risks of sleep 'problems' in particular (Dement with Vaughan 2000).

Behind these trends and developments, however, lies a further story regarding the advent of the sleep 'clinic', if not the birth of 'sleep medicine'; itself, as we shall see, a contentious or contested term. Self-proclaimed 'landmarks' here, according to the likes of Dement (2000) and other leading authors in the sleep science/sleep medicine field, include the following:

(i) the 'discovery' of sleep apnoea in 1965 (the term 'discovery' is used advisedly given many previous observations and literary precursors to this and other sleep 'disorders', including references by Shakespeare and Dickens, see, for example, Chapter 1);

(ii) the formation of the Association of Sleep Disorder Centres in 1975, subsequently renamed the American Sleep Disorders Association;

(iii) the formation of the patient sleep disorders organisation the American Narcolepsy Association in the same year (1975);

(iv) the publication of the Association of Sleep Disorder Centres and the Association for the Psychophysiological Study of Sleep (subsequently renamed the Association of Professional Sleep Societies), *Diagnostic Classification of Sleep Disorders* in 1979, now superseded by the new *International Classification of Sleep Disorders*, last revised in 1997[3];

(v) the introduction of continuous positive airways pressure (C-PAP) techniques for the treatment of obstructive sleep apnoea syndrome (OSAS) in the 1980s;

(vi) the publication of sleep medicine's first handbook *Principles and Practice of Sleep Medicine* in 1989, soon to be in its fourth edition (Kryger et al 2005); and

(vii) finally, the formation by statute of the National Centre on Sleep Disorders Research (NCSDR) as part of the National Heart, Lung and Blood Institute of the US National Insititutes of Health in the 1990s – the mandate of which is to 'supplement research, promote educational initiatives and co-ordinate sleep-related activities throughout various branches of the US government' (Dement 2000: 12).

The latter, in turn, led to the development of a large project dealing with various aspects of sleep disorders and the establishment of awards to develop educational materials at all levels of training (Dement 2000: 13).

To this 'official' history, we may add the following key factors:

(i) the first clinical description of narcolepsy as an independent disease entity in the 1880s by Gelineau (see Chapter 1 in this book), and the ensuing debate as to its nature, status and treatment, particularly in the 1930s (see, for example, Adie 1926, Camp 1907, Levin 1934), with a further clinical revival or re-creation of the condition in the late 1960s and early 1970s;

(ii) the publication of the first scientific paper on REM in 1953 (again see Chapter 1);

(iii) the early applications, in the US at least, of REM research within the psychiatric domain;

(iv) the formation of the Association for the Psychophysiological Study of Sleep in the early 1960s, which brought many sleep researchers together and laid the foundations for the later migration from the sleep *lab* (where basic research on the nature and mechanisms of 'normal' sleep predominated) to the sleep *clinic* (in which sleep 'pathologies' predominate)[4];

(v) the reorientation and re-tooling of sleep research and the sleep lab from the late 1960s onwards – thanks to insomnia and its connections with drug use and dependency – around the costs, safety and efficacy of sleeping pills and prescription hypnotics as a significant public health issue[5]; and

(vi) the further shift of focus or emphasis, from the 1980s onwards, towards sleep apnoea, *qua* disorder of breathing during sleep, as a 'major public health problem' (see for example Phillipson 1993), which in turn consolidated the transition from the sleep lab to the sleep clinic, of which more below.

Much of this, it is apparent, is American in origin. 'Sleep medicine', indeed, to the extent one may speak in such terms, is first and foremost an American 'invention', comprising a variety of interests, which is still, relatively speaking, in its infancy. Certainly great claims are being made about its growth and evolution in the USA at the present time, including a huge push by the Association of Professional Sleep Societies (APSS) to get sleep on the medical curriculum. We can get some measure or sense of these developments in recent times, for instance, and the hype and hyperbole that goes with them, through comparing and contrasting the contents of the first and third editions of the aforementioned handbook, *Principles and Practice of Sleep Medicine* (Kryger et al 2000a). The foreword to the third edition, for example – written, tellingly enough, by the Director of the Division of *Lung Disease*, National Health, Lung and Blood Institute – pays particular tribute to the book as the 'primary resource' for the field of sleep disorders medicine, noting *inter alia*: (i) the 'amazing' amount of revision required between 1989, 1994 and 2000; (ii) the fact that 30 years ago much of this information 'did not exist'; (iii) that some 40 million Americans and millions of others around the world suffer some type of sleep disruption or sleep disorder, with numbers still growing; and (iv) that sleep disorders are a 'true public health problem' (Kiley 2000: xvii). Research advances over the years, Kiley claims, have 'opened the eyes of the medical community to the importance of sleep to health and productivity'. Within this time span, moreover, sleep disorders, once an 'experimental venture', have become 'increasingly recognized and accepted within many spheres of medicine. This, in part, is due to a more thorough understanding of the etiology of common sleep disorders and the introduction of new treatments with the *promise of more interventions on the horizon*' (2000: xvii). 'Today', it is concluded, 'we can safely say with confidence that *sleep disorders medicine is a real medical discipline, grounded in science and worthy of the respect and attention of the entire medical community*'. 'Much remains to be done', nonetheless, it is conceded, in order to 'meet the many needs and opportunities of the field' (2000: xvii).

The preface by the editors adopts an equally eulogising or proselytising tone, noting how the knowledge base 'keeps growing', and how the book is 'very different' from the first edition, including not simply more chapters (from 95 to 110) but 45 entirely new ones (i.e. new topics or new authors). 'New knowledge and new conditions', it is claimed, 'have superseded topics that seemed important a decade ago'. Sleep medicine, indeed, is hailed as a 'model of diversity' – including pulmonologists, neurologists, psychiatrists, psychologists, internists, otolaryngologists, primary care providers and dentists (Kryger et al 2000b: xxi). A paediatric companion volume, moreover, *Principles and Practice of Sleep Medicine in the Child* (Ferber and Kryger 1995), has also been produced, justified on the grounds that most paediatricians surveyed wanted their own book (Kryger et al 2000b: xxi) and that although 'nominally many of the same sleep disorders are seen in both children and adults (for example, sleepiness and sleep-associated breathing abnormalities), the presentations, diagnoses and treatments are quite different in the two groups (Ferber and Kryger 1995: Preface).

There has, quite clearly, been an enormous expansions of sleep (disorder) clinics in recent years, particularly in America. Membership of the American Academy of Sleep Medicine has more than doubled since 1993 from just over 2,200 to nearly 4,900, whilst the number of *accredited* facilities for treating sleep disorders, according to recent American Academy of Sleep Medicine figures, has jumped from 3 in 1978 to 678 in 2003. Nearly two thirds of this growth, indeed, has occurred since 2000 alone (Norbutt 2004).

Opportunities abound, moreover, for the entrepreneurial or enterprising physician to move in on this expanding market. Norbutt (2004), for example, in a tellingly entitled article 'waking up to sleep clinics: growing industry offers eye-opening opportunities', published in *American Medical Association News*, makes no bones about this. Increasing acknowledgement of the risks of sleep problems and increasing acceptance of sleep medicine, he argues, have resulted in more referrals to sleep clinics in the United States than ever before – almost 40% now are from primary care physicians. This has provided doctors, for the first time, with the opportunity to make a 'ground-flooring investment in a sleep clinic'. Most health care insurers moreover, it appears, including Medicare and Medicaid programmes, cover investigation and treatment at sleep centres with advanced certification (Norbutt 2004). Companies too, apparently, are now seeking physician partnerships in new facilities. One doctor for example, it is reported, recently opened a clinic in Dayton Ohio as a joint venture with Sleepcare Diagnostics, a growing company based in nearby Madison Ohio (Norbutt 2004).

But what, exactly, is being treated in these new found or new fangled clinics? The answer, as already noted, is not insomnia – the most common sleep-waking complaint – it is instead sleep apnoea. Officially 'discovered' in 1965, sleep apnoea has emerged as a far more robust or reliable problem for sleep clinicians than the shifting sands of insomnia, allowing 'sleep medicine' to break away from its early psychiatric moorings and move into the mainstream (Kroker 2005). Here, moreover, is a sleep disorder that can, effectively, be measured, monitored, diagnosed and treated in a sleep clinic, with little or no reference to the patient's own subjective reports or awareness of the problem: a shift, that is to say, from subjective *symptoms* to objective *signs* in which irresistible sleepiness is recast as a breathing disorder in sleep (Kroker 2005). Whilst insomnia, in short, has always been a self-diagnosis, sleep apnoea requires the intervention and interpretation of the expert sleep clinician (Kroker 2005): a marriage made in heaven?

These developments are supported or fuelled by a range of facts and figures regarding this newly emergent disorder. Sleep apnoea, for example, is said to be a major cause of excessive daytime sleepiness (EDS) and associated health problems, including heart attacks and strokes, thus providing a staple diet, alongside conditions such as narcolepsy, for the sleep clinic. It is also deemed to be a major risk factor as far as accidents on the roads are concerned, given its prevalence amongst truck drivers. Epidemiological estimates, indeed, indicate the condition is most common in the 40–65 age group, with prevalence around 4% (3–8%) in men and 2% in women (Partinen and Hublin 2000). Among obese subjects, hypertensives and some other patient groups, however, these prevalence rates rise significantly; a fact of no small importance given that approximately 60% of Americans are thought to be either overweight or clinically obese. 'Tackling severe sleep apnoea', moreover, as one sleep disorders specialist puts it, 'makes controlling obesity easier'; part and parcel, he claims, of 'good medicine today' (quoted in Norbut 2004). With sleep apnoea cited as the most common reason for referral to a sleep medicine specialist (NSF 2000), and an estimated 80% of people with sleep apnoea still undiagnosed in the States, the potential for clinical expansion is huge[6].

A related trend, worthy of comment in this context, concerns the growing evidence linking children's sleep problems with behavioural and emotional problems, including conditions such as Attention Deficit/Hyperactivity Disorder (ADHD). Part of the problem, it is claimed, as far as conditions such as ADHD are concerned, may lie with undiagnosed sleep-related breathing disorders such as sleep apnoea, which in turn disrupt children's sleep, causing daytime fatigue, hyperactivity and inattention. The irony here, as Martin (2003: 233) comments, is that the very treatment of ADHD through Ritalin (an amphetamine-like stimulant) may actually exacerbate the problem as far as any underlying sleep disorder is concerned creating a vicious circle.

'Remedies' or 'prescriptions' for sleep problems nonetheless are many and varied, depending on the nature and severity of the problem in question, both inside and outside the clinic. These, as touched on earlier, range from the '*judicious* usage' of *prescription hypnotics* – justified by leading authorities such as Dement on the grounds that past problems of barbiturates and benzodiazepines have now in large part been overcome through a new class of safer, more effective hypnotics known as Imidazopyridines (e.g. Ambien) (Dement with Vaughan 2000: 163) – and *sedating anti-depressants*, to *continuous positive airways pressure (C-PAP)*; *cognitive behavioural therapy* and *parenting skills,* to *over-the-counter remedies and self-medications* (such as Nytol or Sleep-Eez), *alternative therapies* (such as hypnosis, biofeedback, acupuncture, herb and flower remedies), *self-help books* and on/off-line *support groups.*

Equally interesting here, in the context of broader healthicising trends, are the latest calls, cast within an educational, self-empowering mould, for basic principles of 'sleep hygiene'. Sleep hygiene, as we saw in Chapter 2, is far from a new or novel idea: it has a long if not illustrious history, from the ancient Greek regimen, through late Renaissance references (Dannenfeldt 1986) to popular early twentieth century texts such as Edmund Jacobson's (1938) *You Can Sleep Well: The ABCs of Restful Sleep for the Average Person.* It is, however, being *increasingly* seized upon, pushed or touted in the current era where claims of chronic sleep deprivation and its risks to public health and safety abound. People, it is argued, should 'take responsibility for educating themselves about sleep' (Dement with Vaughan 2000: 15), including principles and practices of sleep hygiene which, it is claimed, need scheduling into their lives in the name of health, happiness and well-being. The simple goal of 'good sleep hygiene', from this point of view:

> . . . is to do everything possible to foster good sleep at night. Sleep hygiene includes non-psychological elements, such as avoiding caffeine

before bedtime, but *many of the elements are behavioural. Keeping a regular schedule* is one of the most important behaviours for *healthy sleep*. A regular schedule *helps train your sleep cycle* in the same way that running at the same time every morning conditions you to prepare for exercise at that time. Sticking to a regular sleep schedule seven days a week is a sacrifice worth making if it helps you maintain peak condition throughout the week. *Consider it 'doctor's orders'*.

(Dement with Vaughan 2000: 15, my emphasis)

More generally, we are told, sleep medicine has a critical role to play in public health and public policy formation. The challenge sleep specialists now face, it is argued, is to 'participate in the development of comprehensive conceptual paradigms necessary for resolving the social, health and safety issues associated with people getting proper sleep. Such paradigms are essential if the scientific principles of sleep research are to influence public policy positively' (Mitler et al 2000: 581). The 'special expertise of sleep medicine professionals', it is claimed:

> . . . confer a *unique and heightened set of obligations to address and the political influence to shape rational public policy*. Research indicates that sleep, sleepiness and inattention related to sleep loss and biological rhythms adversely affect workers. This, in turn, leads to public health problems and underscores the need for *wiser public policy concerning sleep and sleep disorders*.
>
> (Mitler et al 2000: 586, my emphasis)[7].

These calls in turn are backed up or facilitated by a range of actual and virtual organisations – patient, public and professional – focused on sleep matters. The American National Sleep Foundation, for example, alongside equivalent organisations in other countries such as the British Sleep Foundation (established in 1999), is dedicated to preventing 'catastrophic accidents' caused by sleep deprivation and excessive daytime sleepiness, enhancing quality of life 'for millions who suffer from sleep disorders' and generally improving public health and safety around sleep and sleep disorders, including a range of materials, activities and events, together with guidelines on sleep services and 'getting involved'. To this, we may add many other patient groups and organisations, focused around a broad range of sleep-related problems, issues and pathologies. The Narcolepsy Association UK, for instance, is an association of narcoleptics, their relatives and others interested in 'improving their lot'. This includes 'promoting awareness of narcolepsy', the provision of 'authoritative information', the establishment of local self-help groups, pressing for the recognition of narcolepsy as a disability, encouraging research into its causes and treatment, and co-operating with narcolepsy associations overseas, such as the American Narcolepsy Association (established in 1975).

This may be the *general* state of play as far as relations between sleep, health and medicine are concerned, but instructive comparisons and contrasts may nonetheless be drawn here on either side of the Atlantic. Sleep apnoea, for example, has had a far more difficult time getting established in Britain than in the USA, including critical debates in *The Lancet* and the *British Medical Journal* as to whether or not it is a sleep disorder at all (Shapiro et al 1981), the 'relevance of sleep apnoea to public health' and the effectiveness of C-PAP vis-à-vis other treatment options such as weight loss (see, for example, Wright et al 1997a and the ensuing debate in the *British Medical Journal*: Stradling and Davies 1997, Wright et al 1997b). Views are divided, moreover, regarding the very nature and status of 'sleep medicine', with one camp seeing it as a distinct specialty and another seeing sleep itself as the preserve or province of other medical disciplines such as neurology, psychiatry and so on. The Royal Society of Medicine, for instance, has a 'Sleep Medicine Section', formerly called the 'Sleep and its Disorders Forum', comprising anaesthetists, basic research scientists, clinical pharmacologists, ENT specialists, GPs, health care professionals, neurologists, nurses, occupational medicine physicians, oncologists, respiratory physicians, psychiatrists, psychologists and physiologists. In reality, however, the practise of 'sleep medicine' is dominated by respiratory physicians such as pulmonologists, ENT specialists and other kindred spirits. This, in turn, is reflected in sleep clinic provision. The British Sleep Society (2003), for example, lists a total of 159 sleep clinics/service providers in the UK in 2003 – a mixture of NHS/public, private and university facilities, with 0–18 dedicated beds, many of which, on closer inspection, turn out to be respiratory labs or units primarily tooled or geared up to diagnose and treat sleep (*qua* breathing) disorders such as sleep apnoea. In the UK, indeed, it is the British Thoracic society, in preference to the British Sleep Society, that claims the 'right' to develop sleep training and education (Stanley 2004, personal communication).

As I write, in fact, the British Sleep Alliance – which represents organisations such as Brake, the British Lung Foundation, the British Sleep Society, the British Snoring and Sleep Apnoea Association, the British Thoracic Society, Relate, the Royal College of Physicians, the Royal College of Psychiatrists, the Royal Society for Prevention of Accidents, and the Sleep Apnoea Trust Association – is calling upon Government and the NHS to increase resources for sleep services. The group's 'call for action' urges a more 'proactive approach' to reducing sleep-related morbidity and mortality; greater recognition of the impact of sleep-related disorders; and, the financial resources to supply an 'adequate infrastructure' for the management of excessive sleepiness, which, it is claimed, affects over 3.5 million people in the UK and is a major cause of serious accidents. Untreated obstructive sleep apnoea syndrome, again, features prominently in these calls, including the tabling of a Private Members' Bill on sleep apnoea through the parliamentary working group on sleep disorders.

What we have here, in summary, are a variety of cross-cutting themes and issues, which, taken together, do indeed point toward a growing or increasing medicalisation of sleep in various guises, particularly in the USA; from the ups and downs of prescription hypnotics to the advent of sleep clinics, if not the birth of 'sleep medicine' as a distinct specialty with its own lexicon of sleep disorders, including what looks like its trump card, sleep apnoea. Service provision, to be sure, is still patchy and limited in scope, particularly in the UK, but moves are clearly afoot here to raise the public profile of this problem if not remedy the situation through concerted political efforts on a number of fronts. To this we may add increasing trends towards the healthicisation of sleep, where lifestyle choices and individual responsibility in the interests of good sleep hygiene and the pursuit of sleep-smart habits loom large: a new form of governmentality, one might say, in the name of health, happiness and the wisdom and virtue of a 'well-slept' life. Sleep, as this suggests, elaborating on our earlier discussion, becomes caught up in a tangled web of normality and deviance, health and illness, morality and risk, safety and danger, across the lay–professional divide.

What role do the media play?

Another important question arises at this point, however, in thinking through the 'old' and 'new' faces of medicalisation: what role do the media play in all this? As far as the medicalisation/healthicisation of sleep is concerned, a variety of roles may be discerned or delineated, ranging from (past) media exposés of the dangers of sleeping tablets or pills (Gabe and Bury 1996b), to reports on the risk of being 'overdrawn' at the 'sleep bank' and handy-cum-healthy 'tips' for a 'good night's sleep'. The media, in other words, as in all other spheres of medical interest or intervention, may be enemy or ally, advocate or critic, sponsor or saboteur, when it comes to involvement in sleep-related matters.

Kroll-Smith (2003), for example, in a prescient piece on popular media and excessive daytime sleepiness (EDS), takes as his point of departure the apparent disjuncture between the aforementioned levels of reported sleepiness and the lack of clinical attention to such matters in everyday medical practice. The public, he argues, given this disjuncture, are increasingly advised and informed, encouraged and cajoled by 'extra-local', 'textualised' forms of knowledge or 'textually mediated forms of ruling', cast in the rhetoric of medicine, including newspapers, magazines and the Internet. These very sources, it is contended, provide a pervasive cultural directive to become conscious of soporific states such as EDS *without the direct intervention of clinical medicine* (2003: 626; see also Kroll-Smith 2000).

This, it seems, is a fact not lost on sleep specialists or medics themselves. Dement, for example, reviewing trends in sleep science and sleep medicine, notes how sleep-related information on the Internet, including numerous website pages devoted to sleep and its disorders, provides a *resource* for physicians, patients and the public at large. The average person today, he proclaims, 'knows a great deal more about sleep and its disorders than the average person at the end of the 1980s' (2000: 13). The number of sleep-related websites indeed is truly astounding. Sleepnet.com, for example – established in 1995 with the motto 'Everything you wanted to know about sleep but were too tired to ask' – is a website designed to link all sleep information located on the Internet so as to 'empower the public'. Currently sleepnet.com contains over 80,000 pages with more than 2 million page views per month, including information on 'sleep disorders', 'sleep links', 'forums' of various sorts, not to mention the 'sleepmall' facility with its many sleep-related products for purchase.

At the same time, concerns are being voiced about the quality of some of this information. Much of the lay press attention to sleep today, Dement (2000) argues, is 'superficial and narrow', compared to 'major stories' in the 1990s which raised many 'tough questions' about how to balance round-the-clock operations with the proper sleep and safety of workers. Common features of such articles are deemed to include a 'light treatment' of 'how little sleep we get because of our hectic modern lifestyles' and feature 'simplistic self-help ideas' and 'ask your doctor' suggestions. These superficial articles moreover, Dement continues, often 'underscore the lack of public awareness about the gravity of sleep-related problems'. Health professionals therefore, he concludes, in keeping with his previous pronouncements, must 'assume responsibility for the inadequate information about sleep and sleep problems available to the general public' (2000: 13).

Kroll-Smith (2003), in this context, flirts with a provocative idea, borrowed from the likes of Bauman and Beck. Whilst EDS, rightly or wrongly, is increasingly reported in the media not simply as a symptom but as a distinct disorder in its own right, medicine itself, he argues, given these more porous textualised forms of knowledge and rhetorical forms of authority (authority cast in the rhetoric of medicine, that is to say), is become something of a 'zombie institution' (half dead and half alive): a situation in which past panoptical forms of control increasingly rub shoulders with those of a more post-panoptical nature. Recast in these terms then, the medicalisation and healthicisation debate, sleep-related or otherwise, takes on important new 'extra-medical' and 'extra-institutional' dimensions. The institutional authority of medicine, in other words:

> . . . remains a potent factor in the day-to-day lives of ordinary people, but illuminated in this inquiry into sleep and sleepiness is an alternative authority expressed in the voices of print and digital media. This second,

rhetorical authority, is reaching into the mundane lives of people fash-
ioning what will count as a personal health issue. The idea or culture
of medicine will continue to exert a powerful hold on our lives. But this
power is likely to be more discursive and less personalized than
routinely found in the physician–patient encounter.

(2003: 639)

This, however, is far from the end of the matter as far as sleep and the media
is concerned, particularly the broadcasting media, whose roles extend well
beyond the mere documentation of sleep matters to outright cases of exper-
imentation or manipulation in the name of entertainment. Fly-on-the-wall
programmes on weird and wonderful sleep disorders, in this respect, including night-time recordings of people walking, talking or eating whilst asleep,
are the tip of the iceberg. The recent UK Channel 4 television series
'Shattered', for example, broke new ground in reality-cum-game-show TV:
the Big Brother of Big Brother so to speak. Contestants in this dubious
series willingly underwent a week of sleep deprivation in the hope of win-
ning a maximum total prize money of £100,000, with £1,000 deducted
each time a contestant fell asleep. Each day one dozing contestant was
eliminated, with viewers tuning in each night (or logging on to the
Channel 4 website) in order to see the ill effects of sleep deprivation in
action, so to speak, and to hear the official pronouncements of the two
Shattered sleep experts (a psychiatrist and a sleep disorders specialist): a
vicarious or voyeuristic form of pleasure in the lack of sleep of others, with
spectacular if not obscene qualities. Throughout the contest, the website
carried a range of stories, fact and figures about sleep, updates on contestants' sleepiness and performance, and the opportunity to take part in
an on-line sleep survey. The winner of this fiasco, a bleary-eyed female
trainee police officer, bagged a cool £97,000 having clocked up a total of
179 hours of sleep deprivation. Whatever next?

'Avoiding' or 'resisting' medicalisation/ healthicisation? The management of sleep 'problems' in everyday life

A possible charge that may be leveled at much of the foregoing discussion is that it paints a largely over-drawn picture of these medicalising/
healthicising trends in which 'lay' people are portrayed in largely passive,
uncritical terms, with resistance dismissed as a near impossibility. This, of
course, is far from the case. Medicalisation, as previously stated, is clearly
no one-way street (Conrad 1992). It is instead a complex process – more
often a question of degree, to repeat, rather than an either/or state of affairs
– with many possible roles and relationships between medical and lay
worlds, textually mediated or not, including both active collaboration and

outright rejection or resistance (Giddens 1991; Williams and Calnan 1996). Sleep disruption and sleep problems, in turn, may be normalised in various ways within the lay populace, whilst many alleged sleep disorders, as we have seen, remain undiagnosed and untreated. There are, moreover, as this book surely testifies, many other important chapters to be written on sleep that carry us far beyond these medicalisation/healthicisation debates.

Just as there is a danger of over-doing the medicalisation/healthicisation story, however, there is equally a danger of underplaying it. This is particularly the case when trends, which at first glance look like demedicalisation, turn out, on closer inspection, to be variants on well entrenched themes or cases of remedicalisation/healthisation in new, more all-encompassing *qua* self-empowering guises, including the turn toward alternative and complementary therapies (Lowenberg and Davis 1994).

The wealth of sleep self-help literature, for instance, is a case in point: an overflowing array of advice books and 'expert' guidance, both medical and non-medical, conventional and non-conventional in kind, is ready and waiting for the tired and weary adult or the anxious parent to pluck off the shelf or download from the web. From *The Insomnia Kit* (Idzikowski 1999) for 'those who have become seriously sleepless', to *Solve Your Child's Sleep Problems* (Ferber 1985), and the *No-cry Sleep Solution: Gentle Ways to Help Your Baby Sleep Through the Night* (Pantley 2002); *Learn to Sleep Well*, for 'those sleepers who want to sleep better' (Idzikowski 2000) or *The Good Sleep Guide* (Van Straten 1996) to *'Is My Child Overtired? The Sleep Solution for Raising Happier, Healthier Children* (Wilkoff, 2000); *Sleep: The Easy Way to Peaceful Nights* (Hollyer and Smith 2002), to *Sleeping Like a Baby: A Sensitive Approach to Solving Your Child's Sleep Problems* (Sadeh 2001), *The New Baby and Toddler Sleep Programme* (Pearce and Bidder 1999) and *Helping Your Baby or Child to Sleep* (Welford 1999), the list of titles grows longer by the day/night.

Again what we appear to have here, returning to previous themes, are further 'expert'-led imperatives or 'textually mediated forms of ruling', imparting both conventional and non-conventional wisdom to their sleepless readers, cast in a self-empowerment mould: new forms of governmentality and self-surveillance, as noted earlier, in the name of health, happiness, wisdom, well-being and a life 'well-slept'[8].

But are we still missing something important here? Hislop and Arber (2003c), in their recent empirical work on women, medicalisation and sleep, certainly think so. In a qualitative investigation of women aged 40 and over, they argue that the medicalisation/healthicisation framework, whilst clearly important, fails to encapsulate a complete understanding of how women manage sleep disruption within the social context of their lives. Women's sleep, to be sure, is a particular target of these medicalising/healthicising trends, but by looking inside the world of women's sleep, it is claimed, we uncover a 'hidden dimension' of 'self-directed' personalised activity which plays a key role in women's response to sleep disruption. It is this *personalisation* of sleep management, these authors contend, which is a 'key chapter' in the story of women's sleep. Aimed at:

> ... relieving symptoms of tiredness, poor concentration and irritability so that women can carry out their roles effectively, sleep management at the personalization level involves women taking responsibility for their sleep, as they have always done, through recourse to personal strategies within the home, ranging from taking hot baths and drinking cocoa, to relocating to other rooms or beds. In this context, women manage their sleep alongside the wider spectrum of tasks and routines that comprise everyday life.
>
> (2003c: 820)

These strategies, it is stressed, including both *preventive* measures to offset potential sleep disruption and *responsive* measures to ameliorate disturbance once it occurs, are actively chosen and designed to help improve the quality of women's sleep, and, by association, the quality of their daily lives. Whilst personalised strategies may form the 'core' of these activities, nonetheless, women's sleep management also permeates the cultures of healthicisation and medicalisation through the use of over-the-counter products, alternative therapies and prescription medications (see for example Phelan et al 2002 and Van der Zee 1997)[9]. The management of women's sleep, therefore, from this perspective, is best understood in term of an:

> ... interplay between personalized, healthicized and medicalized strategies, with choice of strategy mediated by individual perceptions of the severity of sleep disruption, family and work constraints, attitudes to alternative products and practices and perceptions of the role of the medical profession and prescription drugs in the treatment of poor sleep.
>
> (Hislop and Arber 2003c: 820)

For many women, it is concluded, sleep management will take place 'exclusively within the domain of personalised strategies without the need for healthist remedies or prescription medication' (2003c: 835). For other women, the availability of non-prescription medications and complementary health interventions provides an 'optional second-level resource when personalized strategies fail' and when 'self-treatment is favoured as an interim stage before medicalization'. Resort to the medical profession for the treatment of sleep disturbance, in other words, in a prevailing healthist culture, is seen as a 'marked response', to be engaged in 'only when other measures have been tried unsuccessfully' and when 'the impact of sleep disturbance poses a serious threat to health and well-being' (2003c: 835). The management of women's sleep thus needs to be seen as comprising a 'core of personalized activities, with links to healthicization and medicalization' which in turn must be seen in relation to 'the social context in which sleep takes place' (2003c: 835).

Here we return full circle, then, to the fact that the medicalisation/healthicisation of sleep is far from the whole story. The management of sleep in everyday/everynight life, health-related or otherwise, is a complex affair with many possible roles, options or strategies, 'personalised' or otherwise[10].

'Undoing/doing away with' sleep: a 'brave new world'?

There is a further dimension to these debates to consider, however: one that takes us from the 'doing' or promotion of sleep to the potential 'undoing' or 'doing away with' it (altogether), temporarily at least. This might sound like some flight of fancy or the realm of science fiction on my part, of which more below, but the possibility is very real if not already with us today, both inside and outside the boundaries of the sleep clinic.

The US military, for example, as we saw in the previous chapter, is well ahead of the game here, as far as combating sleep is concerned, including their trials of the wakefulness-promoting drug Modafinil (Provigil). The potential applications of Modafinil, as this suggests, extend far beyond the clinical treatment of conditions such as narcolepsy[11]. Concerns are already being voiced, from various quarters, about the 'underground' uptake of the drug, and where precisely this might end. *This, to be sure, is still a far cry from eliminating or doing away with sleep altogether*, permanently or otherwise, but some believe that this is not so far-fetched or far off. Melbin, for example, flirts with just such a possibility. Sleep, he notes:

> . . . is a complex array rather than a single entity. Eventually we will unbundle its parts and do away with some of them. Already people keep irregular waking hours . . . . Researchers try to isolate some of sleep's elements and discover what might substitute for each physical recovery, for dreams and so on. They are already investigating the use of specific drugs that may regulate the timetables of certain physiological functions. People want to have the choice of when to sleep and whether to sleep at all. The prospect of dispensing with it is not so far in the future. The feat is within the capability of a culture that learned how to improve fertility in humans, how to prolong their length of life, and how to transplant organs from one body to another, and that now creates new organisms by genetic transfer. A society that can accomplish those things, in which people's attitudes and organisational needs unite to encourage science in the goal, will undo sleep if it wishes
>
> (1989: 133–4).

The techniques of molecular genetics, indeed, are now enabling scientists to identify individual genes involved in controlling sleep, including those that influence our biological rhythms or clocks, particularly our propensity for early morning rising ('larkness') or bedding down late at night ('owlness') (Martin 2003: 127–30). A mass experiment, for example, at the time of writing, is currently underway at the London Science Museum, under the auspices of its 'Live Science' programme, to determine which of us are larks and which are owls (see www.surrey.ac.uk/SBMS/lark-owl/).

Science-fiction writers take us one or more steps further down the line here, albeit with important moral tales to tell. J.G. Ballard's (1992) *Disaster Area*, for instance, contains an essay 'Manhole 69' that revolves around a group of three surgically altered men who try to do without sleep. Persistent consciousness, however, echoing the above concerns, turns out to be the worst nightmare of all; a case of consciousness closing in on itself, resulting in a withdrawn, empty, reflexless state of 'psychic zero'. Nancy Kress's (1993, 1995, 1996) *Beggars' Trilogy*, in a variant on these themes, explores the hate and fear of regular human beings *qua* sleepers towards the sleepless and the supersleepless – genetically modified humans, originally engineered at the Chicago School of Medicine, who are immune to disease, hunger and the need to sleep. When the sleepless, in the last book, finally plot to take over the world and leave regular humans powerless, civilization and the very meaning of the word 'human' hangs in the balance. Read on . . .[12]

Doing away with sleep altogether then, may or may not ever happen: a distant dream for some and a nightmare scenario for others, depending on your perspective (and how well you sleep?). The push to unbundle or unravel the mysteries of sleep, nonetheless, if not to undo sleep itself, continues apace. Whilst few would surely wish to embrace or opt for continuous wakefulness on a permanent basis should it ever become possible, the prospect of further reducing our need for sleep, or doing without it for longer periods than are currently possible, may prove attractive to some, or all of us perhaps at some times in our lives. Designer sleep for a designer age? Who knows?

Profiting from sleep (problems): commercialisation, consumption and the 'dormant' marketplace

It would be easy to conclude matters here. There is, however, a final dimension to these debates, implicit in much of the foregoing discussion, which, to put it bluntly, boils down to one simple fact: that sleep, in one way or another, is 'big business'. We have a 'dormant' marketplace, in effect, of ready-made consumers, *qua* sleepers, who are catered to and capitalised upon by something akin to a 'sleep industry'. Whether it is sleep or wakefulness, indeed, capitalism profits.

One of the main drivers and beneficiaries of these processes, of course, as far as the medical and health-related aspects of this dormant marketplace are concerned, is the pharmaceutical industry, which quite literally profits from our sleep problems, in keeping with many other ailments and afflictions. Ambien (Zolpidem tartrate), for example, a new (non-benzodiazepine) class of hypnotic produced by Sanofi-Synthelabo Inc., is now the most prescribed sleep medication in the United States. 'Don't underestimate the importance of a FULL night's sleep', the Group's product website proclaims: 'Ambien "works like a dream"' (www.ambien.com). But whose dream are we really talking about here: the shareholders perhaps? Consolidated sales worldwide of Ambien in 2003 amounted to some 1,345 million euros. Demand for Ambien in the United States remains, Sanofi-Sythelabo Inc. report, with prescriptions up 13.4% in 2003, coupled with a 'favourable price effect' (Sanofi-Sythelabo Inc 2004). The market for Cephalon's new wakefulness-promoting drug Modafinil (Provigil) also looks 'healthy' and set for expansion (Cephalon 2004), particularly now it has been approved in the US by an advisory panel to the FDA for the treatment of 'shift-work sleep disorder' and obstructive sleep apnoea (www.modafinil.com).

To this we may add booming sales of over-the-counter products, such as Nytol and Sominex, not to mention combination herbal remedies such as Peaceful Night, Natrasleep, Sleepeaze, Nodoff, mildly sedative herbs such as valerian, camomile, kava kava, passion flower, lemon balm and American skullcap, and other alternative products, such as soporific CDs, self-help books and the like. Even the wisdom of Zen, it seems, is now being marketed and sold on the Internet and in bookstores as the promise of 'enlightenment for a good night's rest' (Chiles 2003). Again, the profits to be made here are huge. Americans, for example, according to the Consumer Health Care Products Association, paid a total of $117 million in 2002 for over-the-counter sleeping aids in 2002 (up from £108 million the previous year): a figure, it should be emphasized, which does not include the purchase of herbal remedies and other alternative products, let alone self-help books.

The product range, as this suggests, is truly astounding: a dizzying array of choices and options, in fact, both conventional and non-conventional, Eastern and Western, for us to take up or tap into. REM™ Dreamline™ products, for example, inspired by Idzikowski's (2000) book *Learn to Sleep Well*, can be found in the 'Healthy Living' area of all major Boots stores, and are also available on the Boots website (www.boots.com) as well as the neuronic 'sleep specialists' website (www.neuronic.com). These products, it is claimed – from floating tanks to yawn mist, bed socks to water beds, sleep suits to drowsy drops, dream baths to beauty sleep products – help you 'wind down after a day of modern living' by 'pampering and comforting' you so that you go to bed feeling 'relaxed and tranquil'. All products are 'sensuous' and have 'aromas that folklore suggests are conducive to sleep' (e.g. lavender). Some products can be used on traditional sleep- and wake-associated acupressure points. Others may be used to massage oneself or one's partner. Many have an impact on body temperature, which affects both sleep onset and sleep quality. The range, moreover, can be used to develop routine and rituals that can help sleep. All in all, we are told, these products prepare your 'body, mind and soul for restful REM sleep': a small *price* to pay, perhaps, for a sound night's sleep?

'Beauty sleep' is another lucrative market or money-spinner which, unsurprisingly perhaps, is particularly targeted at women. Professional 'salon' houses such as Decleor, Gatineau and Elemis, for example, heavily promote their night-time skin care ranges through appeals to the biological functions of sleep and its effects on skin tone and condition. A promotion for Decleor's 'Soin Du Soir', for instance, reads: 'Let your face cream work while you sleep . . . enabling it to repair and replace the damage caused by external elements during the daytime'. Gatineau's 'Laser Night Concentrate', too, we are told, will 'help to stimulate cellular renewal while you sleep', whilst the 'Absolute Night Cream' from Elemis can 'do its energizing work while you sleep' (Williams and Boden 2004). Not content to stop here, companies are also now experimenting with make-up that can be worn overnight, without any damage to the skin, so that you can look your best 24 hours a day – in the bedroom as well as the boardroom!

Perhaps the most obvious sleep-related product or device, however, is the bed which, like all other products in this dormant marketplace, comes in many shapes and sizes – from single beds to double beds, orthopaedic beds to water beds, king-sized beds to bunk-beds, to say nothing of sofa-beds, sleeping bags and futons. In Greater London alone, the number of beds purchased in any one year is estimated to be around 321,000 (Hind 1997). This may sound impressive, but changing consumers' attitudes towards beds, or perhaps, more correctly, increasing consumers' awareness of the need for bed changing, is a major goal of the bed industry. The Sleep Council, for instance, a UK-based organisation offering advice and information for the UK market, places particular emphasis on the marketing of beds on behalf of bed manufacturers and retailers (www.sleepcouncil.com). The aim, we are told, is to create a 'climate for better bed selling' which includes *elevating the bed in consumers' minds as a desirable purchase*' and 'achieving and maintaining general consumer acceptance of a 10-year lifespan for a bed'. Incidentally, March was National Bed Month, in case you missed it!

To beds, of course, we should add bedding and nightwear, including pillows, pyjamas, dressing gowns and other (sexy) garments: items for which the cash till is constantly ringing in high-street stores the length and breadth of the country. Some of these products, to be sure, are more luxurious or ludicrous than others. The 'Sound Asleep' pillow, for instance, invites you to 'nestle down in a supremely comfortable pillow . . . and drift off to your favourite sounds'. 'Buried deep in this pillow', we are told, are 'twin micro speakers offering you high quality private listening'. This, 'innovative set', moreover, 'includes a specially compiled tape of relaxing music – to lull you into the land of nod'. Aaaah . . .

The bedroom has also become a prime target for interior design, with inspirational ideas found in glossy magazines and TV make-over programmes; yet another facet of stylized living or conspicuous consumption perhaps, with or without eco-friendly bedroom furniture.

This, however, is far from the end of the story. Sleep is also, of course, vicariously consumed or enjoyed in a variety of ways for its pure entertainment value, including novels, films, TV programmes and the like in which dormant facts and fictions feature as main or subsidiary themes. Jonathan Coe's (1997) novel *The House of Sleep*, for example, is a recent case in point, alongside other films and dramas where sleep or sleep disorders, dreams or nightmares form part of the storyline, from Disney's *Sleeping Beauty* to Oliver Sack's (1990/1973) *Awakenings*[13], Bram Stoker's (1993/1897) *Dracula* to *Nightmare on Elm Street*. Sleep, in this respect, is fast becoming a box office hit or bestseller: the perfect bedtime reading or viewing one might say. The recent Channel 4 'Shattered' contest, moreover, as noted earlier, marks a new departure in TV entertainment whereby sleep deprivation is turned into a game show: a media spectacle or obscene object of voyeuristic pleasure.

As we saw earlier, companies are also striving to take sleep seriously within the workplace, including the provision of napping rooms and experiments with duvet days. Hollywood too, it seems, is catching on (if not setting the trend) through celebrity contracts for regular shut-eye. When celebrities talk numbers these days, a recent *Sunday Times* article proclaims:

> . . . they're not talking million dollar fees. They're talking hours of sleep. Penelope Cruz, the latest *celebrity sleeper*, recently boasted about a 12-hours-a-night habit, and several of her Hollywood colleagues are said to demand that sleep, or at least no early-morning calls, be *written into their contracts*.
>
> (Kirwan-Taylor 2001, my emphases)

It is tempting, indeed, to conclude here that sleep is not simply being commercialised and capitalised upon, but contracted for or *fetishised* in various ways, in certain segments of (American) society at least: a speculative note to end up perhaps but a provocative one nonetheless as far as the 'well-slept' consumer-cum-citizen is concerned.

Conclusions

Taking as our point of departure the apparent disjunction between the supposed 'epidemic' of sleep problems and disorders in our midst today, and the lack of clinical attention to these matters in everyday medical practice to date, a number of conclusions can be drawn as far as the medicalisation/healthicisation of sleep is concerned.

The medicalisation/healthicisation of sleep, it is clear, is a complex, multi-layered, multi-level process involving a variety of cross-cutting if not contradictory strands, including the changing fate or fortunes of prescription hypnotics, the 'birth' of sleep medicine, the development of an international classification of sleep disorders, lobbying and claim-making regarding sleep and public health, and the growing emphasis on the 'well slept' individual, citizen or society, leading to new forms of governmentality and consumerism in the name of health, happiness and well-being.

This, of course, is not all bad news. The medicalisation of most problems, in fact, usually involves *gains* as well as *losses*. The medicalisation/healthicisation of sleep is no exception. There are, moreover, as we saw in Chapters 1 and 2 in this book, important historical precursors here as far as the medicalisation of sleep is concerned, particularly in the nineteenth century. The social construction of sleep 'problems' or 'pathologies' over time, in this respect, is an important part of the picture. The latter part of the twentieth century, nonetheless, has been particularly significant, as the foregoing discussion suggests: an era in which the social construction of sleep problems or pathologies as a significant risk to public health and safety, and rallying calls for doctors and society to take sleep matters seriously, have been brought to the fore.

What is also worth stressing, perhaps, as far as the 'birth' of sleep medicine and the medicalisaton of sleep is concerned, are the various shifts and transitions underpinning these developments, from the sleep *laboratory* to the sleep *clinic*, and from basic research on the measurement and mechanisms of 'normal' sleep to questions of sleep 'pathologies'. The current concern with sleep apnoea, moreover, throws into critical relief another important feature of 'sleep medicine' today: namely, its power or potential to bypass patient subjectivity and symptomatology altogether in favour of other more objective signs of sleep disorders whilst the patient is asleep (Kroker 2005). Patients, indeed, may very well have a sleep disorder without knowing about it, which in turn legitimises the rationale for the sleep clinic and consolidates the dream or myth of biomedical objectivity (Kroker 2005); an intriguing possibility and a prime opportunity for the enterprising physician.

To this complex picture of cross-cutting influences, we may add the increasingly critical roles of the media and the pharmaceutical industry. The social construction of excessive daytime sleepiness in the media, for example, clearly illustrates the 'textual', 'extra-medical', 'extra-institutional' dimensions of the medicalisation/healthicisation of sleep in the late or post-modern age. At the very least, the media may *amplify* certain problems and issues in this way through cultural directives to become aware of the risks of various somnolent states (cf. Kroll-Smith 2003). The development and marketing of new sleep and wakefulness-promoting drugs, likewise alerts us to the growing power and force of the pharmaceutical industry as a *driver* and *beneficiary* of these processes over time. The management of sleep 'problems' in everyday/everynight life, nonetheless, encompasses a variety of options, some more medicalised or healthicised than others. The med-icalisation/healthicisation of sleep, in other words, is far from the whole story: there are indeed many other important chapters to be written on sleep, both past and present.

As for the huge profits to be made from sleep, these, as we have seen, extend far beyond the medical and health-related aspects of the 'dormant' marketplace, to a variety of other products, 'goods' and services sold and consumed in the name of (a sound, silent or luxurious night's) sleep. Sleep, as this suggests, is now big business, with a burgeoning sleep industry ready and waiting to capitalize upon it. The tension or contradiction between the 'incessant' demands of the so-called 24/7 era and our continuing need to sleep, from this viewpoint, is more apparent than real: capitalism cashes in both ways as 'disrupter' and 'guarantor' of our sleep.

Let me, however, throw a further idea into the melting pot for discussion and debate: an afterthought or postscript if you like. Could it be that what I have been describing here is in fact part and parcel of a far broader set of processes which, for want of a better, less clumsy or cumbersome term, we might refer to as the *'sleepicisation'* of society? That is to say, is there a heightened social awareness and cultural sensitivity to sleep-related matters, which itself, in part, is a response to, or rebuttal of, the 'incessant'/'poorly' slept society? The sleepicisation of society, from this viewpoint, aided and abetted by the media, has the power or potential to permeate all spheres and spaces of society, and to translate all manner of social and medical 'problems' into sleep-related matters. We may even, dare I say it, talk here of the sleepicisation of sociology itself, of which I no doubt stand accused: something to sleep on perhaps?

Notes

1 Doctors are still gatekeepers for medical treatment, Conrad (2004) argues, but their role has become subordinate in the expansion and contraction of medical-ization. The definitional centre of medicalisation, in this respect, 'remains con-stant', but the availability of new pharmaceutical and potential genetic treatments are increasing drivers for new medical categories. Clarke and colleagues' (2003) analysis of the transition from medicalisation to biomedicalisation, however, is too broad brush and conceptually all encompassing, in Conrad's view, thereby losing sight of medicalisation itself (Conrad, personal-communication).

2 The distinction between 'hypnotics' and 'anxiolytics' is a semantic rather than a pharmacological one, which raises the possibility that doctors and/or patients use these drugs in more than one way.

3 Sleep disorders, for ICSD purposes (Diagnostic Steering Committee of the American Sleep Disorders Association 1997), are commonly grouped into: (i) *dyssomnias*, which are disorders of initiating or maintaining sleep and the disorders of excessive sleepiness (such as insomnias and hypersomnias of various kinds, narcolepsy and obstructive sleep apnoea syndrome); (ii) *parasomnias*, which are disorders that do not primarily cause a complaint of insomnia or excessive sleepiness (such as sleep walking, sleep talking, nightmares, sleep paralysis, sleep bruxism); (iii) *sleep disorders* associated with medical or psychiatric disorders (which range from conditions such as sleeping sickness [see below] and fatal familial insomnia [FFI] to chronic obstructive pulmonary disease and sleep-related gastro-oesophageal reflux, and from psychoses and mood disorders to panic attacks and alcoholism); and finally perhaps most intriguingly of all (iv) *proposed sleep disorders* (such as short sleeper, long sleeper, menstrual-associated and pregnancy-associated sleep disorder), which are defined as disorders for which there is 'insufficient information' to confirm their acceptance as definite sleep disorders – a category required, it is claimed, because of the 'rapid advance of sleep medicine that resulted in the discovery of several new sleep disorders' (Thorpy 2000: 547; see also Shapiro 1994). 'Sleeping sickness' is included in the third category above, we are told, 'because this disorder is commonly seen in Africa (*trypanosomiasis*) although it rarely occurs in other continents' (trypanosomiasis is a parasite-borne endemic disease). *Encephalitis lethargica*, on the other hand, often called 'sleepy sickness', is not included 'because it is so rare' (Thorpy 2000: 553), since the great epidemic in the 1920s. See also note 13 below.

4 There are in fact a number of international sleep societies, founded in the last quarter of the twentieth century, including the European Sleep Research Society (ESRS) established in 1971, the Japenese Society for Sleep Research, established in 1978, the Belgian Association for the Study of Sleep (BASS) established in 1982, the Scandinavian Sleep Research Society (SSRS) established in 1985, the Latin American Sleep Society (LASS) established in 1986 and last, but not least, the British Sleep Society, established in 1989 (Thorpy 1991: xxxiii).

5 The first use of the sleep laboratory to evaluate sleeping pills was the 1965 study by Oswald and Priest. See also Oswald (1968) and studies by Kales and colleagues (Kales 1969; Kales and Kales 1970; Kales et al 1969) in the US, which helped establish the role of the sleep laboratory in the evaluation of hypnotic efficacy (Dement 2000; 9). For other commentaries, critiques and observations on sleeping pills and medical practice over time see the (US) Institute of Medicine (1979) report, Smith (1979), Hartman (1979), Morgan (1987), Gabe and Bury (1996b), Speaker (1997), Abraham (1999), Gabe (2001) and Holdbrook (2004).

6 The links between obesity and obstructive sleep apnoea amongst children are also an area of increasing concern, not simply in terms of health, but also in terms of social and educational achievement. There is, furthermore, growing evidence that 'poor sleep' or 'short nights' can disrupt levels of the key hormones in the body that regulate appetite, thereby increasing the risk of obesity.

7 An obvious example of these principles in practice is to be found in (1993) *Wake Up America: A National Sleep Alert* by the National Commission on Sleep Disorders Research.

8 Some on-line self-help sources and support groups are also highly medicalised; see, for example, www.sleepdisorders.com.

9 Most purchasers of over-the-counter sleep aids in Phelan and colleagues' (2002) study were women. The use of sleep aids also rose with age and many purchasers reported 'long-standing sleep problems'. A potential problem of 'inappropriate use' (in relation to the licensed indications of these products and treatment duration), was identified by these researchers amongst nearly half of survey respondents.

10 For a further debate on these issues, see Williams (2004) and Hislop and Arber (2004).

11 In addition to the clinical treatment of nacolepsy, Modafinil is currently used to treat Alzheimer's disease, Attention-Deficit/Hyperactivity Disorder (ADHD), multiple sclerosis-induced fatigue, age-related memory decline, idiopathic hypersomnia and everyday cat-napping. It has also recently received FDA approval in the United States for the treatment of 'shift work sleep disorder' and obstructive sleep apnoea (www.modafinil.com).

12 Other literature in which such themes arise include, for example, Jonathan Coe's (1997) novel *The House of Sleep*, which features a mad sleep scientist hell bent on eliminating it, and Gabriel Garcia Marquez's (1970/1967) *One Hundred Years of Solitude*, where a plague of insomnia descends and people's memories are slowly erased, though later, thankfully, restored through the timely arrival of a gypsy with a magic potion. The real-life equivalent of this, of course, is fatal familial insomnia (FFI), an inherited disorder in which sleep is severely disrupted and death invariably follows. See note 3 above.

13 Sack's (1990/1973) novel provides a moving account of a group of twenty patients – survivors of the great 'sleeping-sickness' or 'sleepy-sickness' (*encephalitis lethargica*) epidemic that swept the world in the 1920s – and the 'awakening' effect they experienced, albeit briefly, some forty years later through a new drug (L-DOPA), administered by Sacks. Recent cases of the disease have been reported and it is now thought to be associated with a particular strain of streptococcal infection. See also note 3 above.

Conclusions: remaining questions and the challenges ahead

The job of this conclusion, in many ways, is already done thanks to the conclusions drawn at the end of each chapter. Rather than restate or repackage them again, therefore, I will take these conclusions as read and focus instead on some remaining questions or meta-themes as a way of drawing this book to a fitting close and of flagging the challenges ahead. To conclude, indeed, may be somewhat premature or misleading, given we are only now just beginning to grapple with this complex and challenging topic following years of oversight or neglect within sociology. This, to repeat, is more than an irony, given that approximately a third of our lives is spent asleep, thereby leaving the sociological task of understanding our lives only two-thirds complete.

What then of these remaining questions or meta-themes?

The first of these returns us to the question raised at the very beginning of the book, namely, whether we need to *reconceptualise* or *rethink* sleep, and if so in what way or ways? The general thrust of this book, as we have seen, taking past sociological neglect and recent emerging interest as its starting point, has been to explore the sociological dimensions of sleep from a variety of angles or vantage points, including sleep and embodiment across the life course, the 'doing' of sleeping in everyday/everynight life, and broader issues concerning the social and cultural patterning of sleep, both past and present, not to mention the dilemmas of sleep or sleeping in late or postmodernity. To the extent that this involves a rethinking or reconceptualisation of sleep, then clearly this has as much to do with sociology itself, given past prejudices and preconceptions, as it does with any other disciplinary claims or approaches to sleep, within or beyond the social sciences. Sleep, moreover, is a complex, multifaceted, multidimensional phenomenon that cannot be reduced to any one domain or discourse, be it biological, psychological, social or cultural. Seen in these terms then, reductionism of any kind must be guarded against whilst simultaneously respecting the discrete analytic potential and irreducible nature of any one of these domains or discourses. Charges of 'imperialist' ambition or intent, in this way, are themselves effectively laid to rest once and for all.

Sociology, in this respect, has much to contribute to an understanding of sleep, both now and in the future, shedding important new light on the social dimensions of sleep, and helping reconfigure existing research agendas in the process. Doing so, in turn, may not simply complement existing research agendas but help redress the current imbalance in sleep research, given its heavy weighting towards basic or clinical questions: a corrective or counterweight of sorts. Sociological approaches to sleep, moreover, as we have seen, raise a series of intriguing problems, puzzles, paradoxes and possibilities, including the changing fate or fortunes if not the 'unravelling' of the sleep role in so-called 24/7 society, the relationship between biological and social 'sleep', the anarchic, anomic, deviant or stigmatised sleeper, to say nothing of the socially attuned or attentive sleeper, the (un)selfish or the (in)considerate sleeper, and the 'undoing', if not the 'doing away with' sleep in various ways, some more dubious than others.

Sleep, as this suggests, involves both voluntary and involuntary, purposive and non-purposive, anonymous/pre-personal and personal/reflexive processes. It is also, to repeat, *embodied* and *embedded* in the social world. This very embodiment and embeddedness, moreover, as Crossley (2004) rightly notes, suggests that sleep has to be negotiated within a dynamic *network*, both actual and virtual, of social influences and social relations (including the potential role of family, neighbourhoods, extended family, employers, education and welfare services and so on), thereby necessitating a 'networked' rather than an atomised or individualised conception of sleep. Sleep, in other words, sociologically speaking, 'takes place' at the intersection of a number of social circles which, despite their distinctiveness, impact mutually upon each other through the mediation of sleep: we 'sleep in social structures' and sleep, in part at least, is 'collective action' (2004: 29). A global perspective on sleep, in turn, serves to remind us of the fitful or fateful, perilous or precarious sleep of people in other war-torn, disease-ridden, famine-stricken parts of the world, and the violations, intended and unintended, of sleep as a basic human right.

These references to sociology's interest or immersion in sleep-related matters, local or global, raise another tricky or awkward question: is a sociology of sleep a contradiction in terms? Much of what I have had to say in this book, the attentive reader will have noticed, concerns what people, lay or expert, say and do about sleep in their conscious waking lives; the meanings, methods, motives and management of sleep or sleeping, that is to say. It may be argued that far from challenging sociology's predominant conscious waking concerns and assumptions, therefore, this simply reaffirms them! Sleep, after all, does involve a loss of waking consciousness. In part, of course, returning to issues raised at the very beginning of the book, this is true. Even if this is conceded, however, it still opens up wholly new areas and avenues of sociological inquiry on *sleep-related matters*, of the kind mentioned above. A sociology of sleep, furthermore, far from precludes a study of actual sleeping bodies, wherever or whenever, nor does it rule out an investigation of the relationship between subjective reports and objective measures of people's sleep. At the most then we are really only talking about a revision or delimiting of our terms of reference, rather than a rejection of them altogether. The division between sleeping and waking life moreover, as we have seen, is far from unproblematic or watertight: a continuum rather than a dichotomy, to all intents and purposes, involving a series of intermediate states between 'deep' sleep and 'alert' wakefulness. The 'recovery' of sleep-related themes and issues in waking life, likewise, further problematises any such neat and tidy division or divide.

This leads us to a third key question: is it a sociology of sleep we are after or something else? On the one hand, a sociology of sleep makes sense, particularly in trying to establish a new and viable domain of study, with the relevant expertise to do so. On the other hand, this may create its own problems or tensions, not least in terms of the risk of 'ghettoising' sleep in one way or another as the province of the marginal or the maverick few, thereby fragmenting the discipline of sociology still further, whilst the real business of sociology grinds on regardless. Sleep, as we have seen, is relevant to most if not all domains of sociological inquiry and social scientific interest. It is not so much a ghettoised sociology of sleep we are after, therefore, but a more general awareness and sensitivity to sleep-related matters within sociology and beyond. Whether or not, of course, this itself is part and parcel of what I have termed the *sleepicisation* of society is a moot point, but it certainly involves a recognition, in these reflexive times, that sleep implicates us all, including us embodied practitioners of our craft as well as those we seek to study.

From here it is but a short step to the related question of multi-disciplinary or inter-disciplinary research. If we are really going to get to grips with sleep in all its richness and glory, then how best are we to do this? The answer, of course, depends on what precisely we are looking at or which questions we are seeking to answer. If, for example, I am solely or simply interested in researching what people think, say or do about sleep in their waking lives, including their attempts to account for the unaccountable (their conscious renderings of the loss of consciousness when asleep, that is to say), then sociology is well placed to do so. If, however, I wish to explore the relationship between the quality or quantity of people's actual sleep and their own subjective reports of their sleep, then some form of collaborative research is probably the best way forward. To the extent, more generally, that we wish to explore the relationship between the biological, psychological, social and cultural dimensions of sleep, then multi-disciplinary or inter-disciplinary research clearly makes sense. *Embodiment* again is a useful *integrating theme* here in any such undertaking or enterprise: a bulwark, in effect, against reductionism of any kind. To speak of inter-disciplinary, or even perhaps trans-disciplinary or post-disciplinary research agendas, nonetheless, may be somewhat premature, given the considerable amount of spadework that still remains to be done *within*, let alone across or beyond, existing disciplinary domains in the social and natural sciences. We should not, moreover, underestimate the vested interests at stake in upholding rather than unravelling the existing division of labour, even in a newly emerging domain such as this one. To do so, indeed, would be not simply conceptually and methodologically, but politically, naive.

The field then, as this suggests, is wide open as far as future agendas and the challenges ahead are concerned, in sociology and beyond. Sociological approaches to sleep may operate on a number of different levels, from the individual/(non)experiential, through the social/interactional to the societal/institutional. Sleep, moreover, is both a rich and fascinating topic in its own right and a new way of seeing or thinking about existing or established sociological research agendas from embodiment to the dilemmas of risk society.

As for the changing fate or fortunes of sleep in late or postmodernity, sleep as we have seen is the source or subject of much concern and claim-making today: part and parcel, indeed, of a broader series of discourses and debates on work time and work ethics, productivity and performance, the public and the private, safety and risk, health and illness, rights and responsibilities. The 'well-slept citizen' or the 'well-slept society', in this respect, may be a more or less distant dream, but either way sleep provides a critical reference point in a changing social world: the last frontier perhaps in an incessant global age, which in true late or postmodern, if not post-dormative, fashion is being done and undone in all manner of ways, for better or worse, including the reframing of the not so humble nap as the smart sleep option or lifestyle choice. To sleep or not to sleep, that is the question: a local and global matter and a shared form of embodied vulnerability that at one and the same time unites and divides us.

References

Abraham, J. (1999) *Therapeutic Nightmare: The Battle of the Worlds most Controversial Sleeping Pill*. London: Earth Scan.

Åckerstedt, T. (1995) Work hours, sleepiness and the underlying mechanisms. *Journal of Sleep Research*. 4 Suppl. 2; 15–22.

Åckerstedt, T. (2004) Sleep – gender, age, stress, work hours, in World Health Organization, Regional Office for Europe *Technical Meeting on Sleep and Health*. European Centre for Environment and Health, Bonn office, Germany (http://www.euro.who.int/noise/activities).

Åckerstedt, T., Arnetz, B.B. and Anderzen, I. (1990) Physicians during and following night call duty – 36 hour ambulatory recording of sleep. *Electroencephalography and Clinical Neurophysiology*. 76: 193–6.

Adams Parker, S. (1862) *Remarks Upon Artificial Teeth*. Birmingham: Cornish Brothers.

Adams Parker, S. (1863) Case studies in dental decay. *British Journal of Dental Science*. VI, 84: 263–8.

Adie, W.J. (1926) Idiopathic narcolepsy. *Brain*. 49: 257–306.

Adler, A. (1912) Dreams and dream interpretation, in *The Theory and Practice of Individual Psychology*, transl. P. Radin. London: Kegan Paul.

Allatt, P. (1996) Conceptualizing parents from the standpoint of children: relationships and transition in the life course, in J. Brannen and M. O'Brien (eds) *Children in Families: Research and Policy*. London: Falmer Press.

Alvarez, A. (1996) *Night: An Exploration of Night Life, Night Language, Sleep and Dreams*. London: Vintage.

Amnesty International (2005) Guantánamo – an icon of lawlessness, 6 January 2005. Amnesty International, AMR 51/002/2005 (www.amnesty.org).

Anthony, C. and Anthony, W.A. (2001) *The Art of Napping at Work*. London: Souvenir Press.

Anthony, W.A. (1997) *The Art of Napping*. New York: Larson Publications.

Arber, S. and Ginn, J. (1995) *Connecting Gender and Ageing: A Sociological Approach*. Buckingham: Open University Press.

Arber, S. Davidson, K. and Ginn, J. (eds) (2003) *Gender and Ageing: Changing Roles and Relationships*. Maidenhead: Open University Press.

Archer, J. (2002) *A Prison Diary Vol. I – Belmarsh: Hell*. London: Pan Books.

Archer, M. (1995) *Realist Social Theory: The Morphogenetic Approach*. Cambridge: Cambridge University Press.

Aristotle (1957) *On the Soul, Parva Naturalia, on Breath* (translated by W.S. Hett). London: Heinemann.

Arksey, H. (1998) *RSI and the Experts: The Construction of Medical Knowledge.* London: Routledge.

Armitage, J. (ed.) (2000) *Paul Virilio: From Modernism to Hypermodernism and Beyond.* London: Sage Publications.

Armstrong, D. (1995) The rise of surveillance medicine. *Sociology of Health and Illness.* 17: 393–404.

Artemidorous of Daldis (1664) *Oneirocritica/The Interpretation of Dreams* (translated by R. Wood, abridged). London.

Aserinsky, E. and Kleitman, N. (1953) Regularly occurring periods of eye motility, and concomitant phenomena, during sleep. *Science.* 118: 273–4.

Aubert, V. and White, H. (1959a) Sleep: a sociological interpretation I. *Acta Sociologica.* 4: 1–16.

Aubert, V. and White, H. (1959b) Sleep: a sociological interpretation II. *Acta Sociologica.* 4: 46–54.

Ayukawa, J. (2003) Night-time and deviant behaviour: the changing night scene of Japanese youth, in B. Steger and L. Brunt *Night-time and Sleep in Asia and the West: Exploring the Dark Side of Life.* London: Routledge Curzon.

Bakhtin, M. (1968) *Rabelais and his World.* Cambridge MA: MIT Press.

Ballard, J.G. (1992) *Disaster Area.* London: Flamingo.

Bataille, G. (1987/1962) *Eroticism* (translated by M. Dalwood). London: Boyars.

Bauman, Z. (1992) *Mortality, Immortality and Other Life-Strategies.* Cambridge: Polity Press.

Baxter, V. and Kroll-Smith, S. (2005) Napping at work: shifting boundaries between public and private time. *Current Sociology.* 53, 1: 33–55.

Bechterev, V.M. (1932) *General Principles of Human Reflexology.* New York: International Publications.

Beck, U. (1992) *Risk Society.* London: Sage Publications.

Beck, U. (2000) *The Brave New World of Work.* Cambridge: Polity Press.

Beevor, A. (1998) *Stalingrad.* London: Viking.

Ben-Ari, E. (1996) From mothering to othering: organization, culture, and nap time in a Japanese day-care centre. *Ethos.* 24, 1: 136–64.

Ben-Ari, E. (2003) Sleep and night-time combat in contemporary armed forces: technology, knowledge and the enhancement of the soldier's body, in B. Steger and L. Brunt *Night-time and Sleep in Asia and the West: Exploring the Dark Side of Life.* London: Routledge Curzon.

Benedict, R. (1989/1946) *The Chrysanthemum and the Sword: Patterns of Japanese Culture.* Boston MA: Houghton Mifflin.

Berger, H. (1930) Ueber das Elekroenkephalogramm des Menschen. *Journal of Psychological Neurology.* 40: 160–79.

Berger, R.J. (1961) Tonus of extrinsic laryngeal muscles during sleep and dreaming. *Science.* 134: 840.

Bernd, E. Jnr (1978) *Relax.* Orlando FL: Grenn Madainn Foundation.

Blake, H., Gerrard, R.W. and Kleitman, N. (1939) Factors influencing brain potentials during sleep. *Journal of Neurophysiology.* 2: 48–60

Blaxter, M. (1990) *Health and Lifestyles.* London: Routledge.

Bliwise, D.L. (1996) Historical change in daytime fatigue. *Sleep.* 19: 462–4.

Bliwise, D.L. (2000) Normal ageing, in M.H. Kryger, T. Roth and W.C. Dement (eds) *Principles and Practice of Sleep Medicine* (3rd edn). Philadelphia/London: W.B. Saunders.

Bonnet, M.H. and Arnaud, D.L. (1995) We are chronically sleep deprived. *Sleep.* 18: 908–11.

Borde, A. (1542) *A Compendious Regiment, or Dietarie of Health.* London.

Bouchard, C. (1886) Sur la theorie les variations de la toxicite urinaire pendant la veille, et pedant le sommeil. *College of the Royal Academy of Science.* 102: 727.

Bourdieu. P. (1984) *Distinction: A Social Critique of the Judgement of Taste.* London: Routledge.

Bourdieu, P. (1990) *The Logic of Practice.* Cambridge: Polity Press.

Bourdieu, P. (2000) *Pascalian Meditations.* Cambridge: Polity Press.

Brannen, J. and O'Brien, M. (eds) (1996) *Children in Families: Research and Policy.* London: Falmer Press.

Brannen, J. and Moss, P. (1988) *New Mothers at Work: Employment and Childcare.* London: Unwin Paperbacks.

Bremer, F. (1935) Cerveau 'isole' et physiologie du sommeil. *Comptes Rendus des Seances de la Société de Biologie et de ses Filiales.* 118: 1235–41.

Brenner, S.O, Levi, L., Salovaara, H., Åkerstedt, T., Hjelm, R., Söbom, D. and Tellenback, S. (1985) Job insecurity and unemployment: effects on health and wellbeing and an evaluation of coping measures, in C. Westcott, P.-G. Svensson and H.F.K. Zöllner. Copenhagen: World Health Organization, Regional Office for Europe.

British Medical Association (2002) *Effects of Sleep Deprivation on Doctors: A Briefing Paper from the Board of Science and Education.* London: BMA (www.bma.org.uk/ap.nsf/Contents/sleepdeprivation).

British Medical Association (2004) *Hospital Doctors – Junior Doctors' Hours.* London: BMA (www.bma.org.uk/ap.nsf/content/hospitaldoctorsjunhrs).

British Sleep Society (2003) *UK and Ireland Sleep Service Providers Directory.* Huntingdon: British Sleep Society.

Brokaw, J., Fullertone-Gleason, L., Olson, L., Crandall, C., McLaughlin, S. and Sklar, D. (2002) Health status and intimate partner violence: a cross-sectional study. *Annals of Emergency Medicine.* 39, 1 (January): 31–8.

Broom, D. and Woodward, R.V. (1996) Medicalisation reconsidered: towards a collaborative approach to care. *Sociology of Health and Illness.* 8: 357–78.

Brown, P. (2001) Ruling puts airport night flights in doubt: widespread action likely after European court backs Heathrow resident's right to enjoy a good night's sleep. *The Guardian.* 3rd October: 10.

Brown-Sequard, C.E. (1889) Le sommeil normal comme le sommeil hypnotique, est le resultant d'une inhibition de l'activate intellectuelle. *Archives de Physiologie Normale et Pathologique.* 1: 333–5.

Browne, A. (2000) How sleep can save your life. *The Observer.* 29th October: 12.

Brunt, L. (2003) Between day and night: urban time schedules in Bombay and other cities, in B. Steger and L. Brunt *Night-time and Sleep in Asia and the West: Exploring the Dark Side of Life.* London: Routledge Curzon.

Brunt, L. (2004) Nightblind: sociology and the study of the urban night. Paper presented at the first ESRC 'Sleep and Society' seminar, 3rd December, University of Warwick.

Bryan, G.S. (1926) *Edison: The Man and His Work*. New York: Garden City Publishing.

Burwell, C.S., Robin, E.D. and Whaley, R.D. (1956) Extreme obesity associated with alveolar hypoventilation. A Pickwickian syndrome. *American Journal of Medicine*. 21: 811–18.

Bury, M. (1997) *Health and Illness in a Changing Society*. London: Routledge.

Bury, M. (2000) Health, ageing and the lifecourse, in S.J. Williams, J. Gabe and M. Calnan (eds) *Health, Medicine and Society: Key Theories, Future Agendas*. London: Routledge.

Camp, C.D. (1907) Morbid sleepiness, with a report of a case of narcolepsy and a review of recent theories of sleep. *Journal of Nervous and Mental Disease*. 2: 9–21.

Campbell, D. (2000) LA homeless sleep in the shadow of wealth. *The Guardian*. 28th December: 14.

Carskadon, M.A., Brown, E.D. and Dement, W.C. (1982) Sleep fragmentation in the elderly: relationship to daytime sleep tendency. *Neurobiology of Aging*. 3: 321–7.

Carvel, J. (2004a) NHS staff in hours crisis. *The Guardian*. 30th July: 1.

Carvel, J. (2004b) Bending the rules for the sake of efficiency – and pay increases for junior doctors. *The Guardian*. 30th July: 4.

Carvel, J., Curtis, P., Glendinning, L. and Sturcke, J. (2004) Hit squads move in as hospitals prepare to deal with limits on working hours: Managers face choice of compromising patient care or failing to meet EU directive. *The Guardian*. 30th July: 4.

Caton, R. (1875) The electric currents of the brain. *British Medical Journal*. 3: 278–82.

Cephalon, Inc. (2004) Cephalon, Inc. reports third quarter financial results (www.cephalon.com).

Chadwick, E. (1997/1842) *Report on the Sanitary Conditions of the Labouring Population of Great Britain* (with a new introduction by D. Gladstone). London: Routledge/Thoemmes Press.

Chiles, E. (2003) *Zen Sleep: Enlightenment for a Good Night's Sleep*. Austin TX: Pilatus Publishing.

Claparede, E. (1905) Esquisse d'une theorie biologique du sommeil. *Archives of Psychology*. 4: 345–9.

Clarke, A., Mamo, L., Fishman, J.R., Shim, J.K. and Fosket, J.R. (2003) Biomedicalization: technoscientific transformations of the health, illness and US biomedicine. *American Sociological Review*. 68 (April): 161–94.

Coe, J. (1997) *The House of Sleep*. London: Penguin.

Cohen, S. and Taylor, L. (1972) *Psychological Survival: The Experience of Long-term Imprisonment*. Harmondsworth: Penguin.

Coleridge, S.T. (1971) *Collected Letters of Samuel Taylor Coleridge, Vol V 1820–25* (edited by E.L. Griggs). Oxford: Clarendon Press.

Coleridge, S.T. (1985) *The Major Works, Including Biographia Literaria*. Oxford: Oxford University Press.

Conrad, P. (1992) Medicalization and social control. *Annual Review of Sociology*. 18: 209–32.

Conrad, P. (2004) The shifing engines of medicalization. Plenary, *British Sociological Association Medical Sociology Group Conference*, 16–18th September, University of York.

Conrad, P. and Leiter, V. (2004) Medicalization, markets and consumers. *Journal of Health and Social Behavior*. 45 extra issue: 158–76.

Conrad, P. and Schneider, J.W. (1980) Looking at levels of medicalization: a comment on Strong's critique of the thesis of medical imperialism. *Social Science and Medicine*. 14: 75–9.

Cooley C.H. (1902) *Human Nature and the Social Order*. New York: Random House.

Coren, S. (1996) *Sleep Thieves: An Eye-opening Exploration into the Science and Mysteries of Sleep*. New York/London: The Free Press.

Cosnett, J. (1997) Charles Dickens and sleep disorders. *Dickensian*. 93, 3: 200–4.

Crick, F. and Mitchison, G. (1983) The function of dream sleep. *Nature*. 304: 111–15.

Crick, F. and Mitchison, G. (1995) REM sleep and neural nets. *Behavioural and Brain Sciences*. 23, 877–82.

Crook, T. (2002) Disciplining sleep: governing the dormant body in nineteenth-century Britain. Paper presented to the Social History Conference, 'Vice and Virtue', University of Manchester.

Crook, T. (2004) Privatising sleep: bodies, beds and civility in Victorian Britain. Paper presented at the first ESRC 'Sleep and Society' seminar, 3rd December, University of Warwick.

Cropley, M. (2004) Rumination and sleep. Paper presented at the British Sleep Society seminar: 'Reconceptualising sleep: the contribution of the social sciences', 15th June, University of Surrey.

Crossley, N. (2001) *The Social Body*. London: Sage.

Crossley, N. (2004) Sleep, reflexive embodiment and social networks. Paper presented at the first ESRC 'Sleep and Society' seminar, 3rd December, University of Warwick.

Culebras, A. (1999) Sleep and narcolepsy. *Archives of Neurology*. 56: 117–18.

Currie, A., Peille, E. and Hanning, C. (2005) Dying for a kip: the importance of sleep medicine. *British Medical Journal Careers*, 330: 53–55.

Czeisler, C.A., Allan, J.S., Strogatz, S.H., Ronda, J.M., Sanchez, R., Rios, C.D., Freitag, W.O., Richardson, G.S. and Kronauer, R.E. (1986) Bright light resets the human circadian pacemaker independent of the timing of the sleep-wake cycle. *Science*. 233: 667–71.

Dana, C. (1884) On morbid drowsiness and somnolence: a contribution to the pathology of sleep. *Journal of Nervous Mental Disease*. 11: 153–76.

Dannenfeldt, K.H. (1986) Sleep: theory and practice in the late Renaissance. *The Journal of the History of Medicine and Allied Sciences*. 41: 415–41.

Davidson, H.C. (1900) *The Book of the Home*. London: Gresham.

de la Mare, W. (1939) *Behold This Dreamer*. London: Faber and Faber.

de Maupassant, G. (n.d.) *The Complete Short Stories of Guy de Maupassant*. London: Blue Ribbon Books.

de Montaigne, M. (1991/1572) *The Complete Essays* (translated by M.A. Screech). London: Penguin.

Deary, I.J. and Tait, R. (1987) The effects of sleep disruption on cognitive performance and mood in house officers. *British Medical Journal* (Clinical Research Education). 295: 1513–18.

Dekker, T. (1969/1609) *The Guls Horne-Booke*. London: Scolar Press.

Dement, W.C. (1976) *Some Must Watch Whilst Others Must Sleep*. New York: Norton.

Dement, W.C. (2000) History of sleep physiology and medicine, in M.H. Kryger, T. Roth and W.C. Dement (eds) *Principles and Practice of Sleep Medicine* (3rd edn). Philadelphia/London: W.B. Saunders.

Dement, W.C. and Kleitman, N. (1957) Cyclic variations in EEG during sleep and their relation to eye movements, body motility and dreaming. *Electroencephalography and Clinical Neurophysiology*. 9: 673–90.

Dement, W.C. with Vaughan, C. (2000) *The Promise of Sleep: The Scientific Connection between Health, Happiness and a Good Night's Sleep*. New York/London: Delacourt Press/Macmillan.

Demetrious, S. (2004) Unsleeping partners. *The Observer*. 28th November, (Living Supplement): 4.

Dennett, D.C. (1978) *Brainstorms: Philosophical Essays on Mind and Psychology*. Montgomery VT: Bradford Books.

Descartes, R. (1971) *Treatise of Man* (French text with translation; commentary by T.S. Hall). Cambridge MA: Harvard University Press.

Descartes, R. (1996/1641) *Meditations on First Philosophy with Selections from Objections and Replies* (edited by J. Cottingham). Cambridge: Cambridge University Press.

Diagnostic Steering Committee of the American Sleep Disorders Association (1997) *The International Classification of Sleep Disorders Diagnostic and Coding Manual*. Rochester MN: ASCA.

Dickens, C. (1909/1836–7) *The Posthumous Papers of the Pickwick Club*. Vol 2. London: Chapman and Hall.

Dickens, C. (1973/1860) *The Uncommercial Traveller and Reprinted Pieces etc.* Oxford: Oxford University Press (Chpt. XIII 'Night Walks').

Dinges, D.F. (1995) An overview of sleepiness and accidents. *Journal of Sleep Research*. 4 (Suppl. 2): 4–14.

Doi, Y. and Minowa, M. (2003) Gender differences in excessive daytime sleepiness among Japanese workers. *Social Science and Medicine*. 56, 4 (Feb): 883–94.

Drugs and Therapeutics Bulletin (2004) What's wrong with prescribing hypnotics? *Drugs and Therapeutics Bulletin*. 42, 12 (December): 89–93.

Dubois, R. (1894) Variations des gaz du sang chez la marmotte rendent l'hibernation en etat de veile et en etat de torpeur. *Comptes Rendus des Seances de la Société de Biologie et de ses Filiales*. 46: 821–3.

Dunier, M. (2000) *Sidewalk*. New York: Farrar, Straus and Giroux.

Duveen, D.I. and Klickstein, H.S. (1955) Antoine Laurent Lavoisier's contribution to medicine and public health. *Bulletin of the History of Medicine*. 29: 164–79.

Dyos, H.J. (1967) The slums of Victorian London. *Victorian Studies*. 11: 5–40.

Ekirch, R. (2001) The sleep we have lost: pre-industrial slumber in the British Isles. *American Historical Review*. April: 343–86.

Elias, N. (1978/1939) *The Civilizing Process Vol. 1: The History of Manners*. Oxford: Basil Blackwell.

Engels, F. (1999/1845) *The Conditions of the Working Class in England* (edited with an introduction and notes by D. McLellan). Oxford: Oxford University Press.

Epstein, R. (1998) Starting times of school: effects on daytime functioning. *Sleep*. 21: 250.

European Court of Human Rights (2001) *Case of Hatton and Others v. the United Kingdom*. 2 October. Strasbourg.

Featherstone, M. and Hepworth, M. (1998) Ageing, the lifecourse and the sociology of embodiment, in G. Scambler and P. Higgs (eds) *Modernity, Medicine and Health*. London: Routledge.

Ferber, R. (1985) *Solve Your Child's Sleep Problems*. London/New York: Dorling Kindersley.

Ferber, R. and Kryger, M. (1995) *Principles and Practice of Sleep Medicine in the Child*. Philadelphia/London: W.B. Saunders.

Feyer, A.M. (2001) Editorials: Fatigue: time to recognise and deal with an old problem. *British Medical Journal*. 322: 808–9.

Firth-Cozens, J. and Moss, F. (1998) Hours, teamwork and stress. *British Medical Journal*. 317: 1335–6.

Fitzgerald, M. and Sim, J. (1979) *British Prisons*. Oxford: Basil Blackwell.

Flanagan, O. (2000) *Dreaming Souls: Sleep, Dreams and the Evolution of the Conscious Mind*. Oxford: Oxford University Press.

Fleming-Michael, K. (2003) The sleep factor. *Soldiers*. (October): 38–41.

Ford, J. (2004) Samuel Taylor Coleridge and 'The pains of sleep', in D. Pick and L. Roper (eds) *Dreams and History: The Interpretation of Dreams from Ancient Greece to Modern Psychoanalysis*. London/New York: Brunner-Routledge.

Foucault, M. (1977) *Discipline and Punish: The Birth of the Prison*. London: Tavistock.

Foucault, M. (1987) *The History of Sexuality, Vol 2: The Use of Pleasure*. Harmondsworth: Penguin.

Foucault, M. (1988) *The History of Sexuality, Vol 3: The Care of the Self*. Harmondsworth: Penguin.

Fox, R.C. (1977) The medicalisation and demedicalisation of American society. *Daedelus*. 106: 9–22.

Freidson, E. (1970) *The Profession of Medicine*. New York: Dodd Mead.

Freud, S. (1976/1900) *The Interpretation of Dreams*. Pelican Freud Library. Harmondsworth: Penguin.

Furman, Y., Wolf, S.M. and Rosenfeld, D.S. (1997) Shakespeare and sleep disorders. *Neurology*. 49: 1171–2.

Gabe, J. (2001) Benzodiazepines as a social problem: the case of Halcion. *Substance Use and Misuse*. 50, 2: 1233–59.

Gabe, J. and Bury, M. (1996a) Risking tranquilliser use: social and cultural perspectives, in S.J. Williams and M. Calnan (eds) *Modern Medicine: Lay Perspectives*. London: UCL Press.

Gabe, J. and Bury, M. (1996b) Halcion nights: a sociological account of a medical controversy. *Sociology*. 45, 1: 447–69.

Gadamer, H.-G. (1996) *The Enigma of Health*. Cambridge: Polity Press.

Gelineau, J.B.E. (1880) De la narcolepsie. *Lancette Franc., Gazette de Hospitaux*. 53: 626–37

Giddens, A. (1991) *Modernity and Self-identity*. Cambridge: Polity Press.

Gilleard, C. and Higgs, P. (2000) *Cultures of Ageing: Self, Citizen and the Body*. London: Prentice Hall.

Gladstone, D. (1997) Introduction, in E. Chadwick *Report on the Sanitary*

Conditions of the Labouring Population of Great Britain. London: Routledge/ Thoemmes Press.

Gleichman, P.R. (1980) Einige soziale Wandlungen de Schlafens. *Zeitschrift fur Soziologie.* 9, 3: 236–50.

Gleick, J. (2000) *Faster: The Acceleration of Just About Everything.* London: Abacus.

Goffman, E. (1961a) *Encounters: Two Studies in the Sociology of Interaction.* Indianapolis IN: Bobbs-Merrill.

Goffman, E. (1961b) *Asylums: Essays on the Social Situation of Mental Patients and Other Inmates.* Harmondsworth: Penguin.

Goffman, E. (1963) *Behaviour in Public Places.* London: Allen Lane.

Goffman, E. (1967) *Interaction Ritual: Essays on Face-to-Face Behaviour.* New York: Doubleday Anchor Books.

Goffman, E. (1981/1963) *Stigma: Notes on the Management of Spoiled Identity.* Harmondsworth: Penguin/Pelican.

Gottlieb, A. (2004) Preface to B. Russell. *In Praise of Idleness.* London: Routledge.

Gray, C.H. (2002) *Cyborg Citizen.* London: Routledge.

Green, C. (1968) *Lucid Dreaming.* London: Hamish Hamilton.

Green, M.J. (1995) What (if anything) is wrong with residency overwork? *Annals of Internal Medicine.* 123: 512–15.

Green, W.E. (1882) Sleepiness, its causes and treatment. *Birmingham Medical Review* XI: 161–74.

Gubrium, J.F. (1975) *Living and Dying at Murray Manor.* New York/London: St Martin's Press/St James Press.

Gubrium, J.F. and Holstein, J.A. (1999) The nursing home as a discursive anchor for the ageing body. *Ageing and Society.* 19: 519–38.

Hall, W.W. (1871) *Sleep or the Hygiene of the Night.* London: James W. Ward.

Hammond, W.A. (1869) *Sleep and its Derangements.* Philadelphia PA: Lippincott.

Haraway, D. (1990) *Simians, Cyborgs and Women.* London: Free Association Books.

Harris, D.F. (1910) *The Physiology and Hygiene of Sleep: Being the Annual Public Lecture on 'The Laws of Health' delivered at the Midland Institute, Birmingham, September 16, 1910.* Birmingham: Cornish Brothers.

Harrison, Y. and Horne, J. (1995) Should we be taking more sleep? *Sleep.* 18, 10: 901–7.

Hartman, E. (1979) *The Sleeping Pill.* New Haven CT/London: Yale University Press.

Hathaway, J.E., Lorelie, A.M., Silverman, J.G., Brooks, D.R., Mathews, R. and Pavlos, C.A. (2000) Health status and health care of Massachusetts women reporting partner abuse. *American Journal of Preventive Medicine.* 19, 4: 302–7.

Haywood, R. (2004) Policing dreams: history and moral uses of the unconscious, in D. Pick and L. Roper (eds) *Dreams and History: The Interpretation of Dreams from Ancient Greece to Modern Psychoanalysis.* London: Brunner-Routledge.

Hearne, K. (1990) *The Dream Machine.* Wellingborough: Aquarian Press.

Henneberg, R. (1916) Über genuine narkolepsie. *Neurol. Zbl.* 30: 282–90.

Hervey, L., Marquis de Saint-Deny (1982/1867) *Dreams and How to Guide Them* (translated by N. Fry). London: Duckworth.

Hess, W.R., Koella, W.P. and Akert, K. (1952) Corticol and subcorticol recordings of anaesthetized cats. Electroencephalography and *Clinical Neurophysiology.* 4: 370–1.

Hilton, B.A. (1985) Noise in acute patient areas. *Research in Nursing and Health.* 8: 283–91.

Hind, J. (1997) London index: beds. *London Evening Standard.* 3rd October.

Hinsliff, G. (2004) Stress becomes the No. 1 complaint of British workers. *The Observer.* 31st October: 9.

Hislop, J. and Arber, S. (2003a) Sleepers wake! The gendered nature of sleep disruption among mid-life women. *Sociology.* 37, 4: 695–711.

Hislop, J. and Arber, S. (2003b) Sleep as a social act: a window on gender roles and relationships, in S. Arber, K. Davidson and J. Ginn (eds) *Gender and Ageing: Changing Roles and Relationships.* Maidenhead/Philadelphia: Open University Press.

Hislop, J. and Arber, S. (2003c) Understanding women's sleep management: beyond medicalization-healthicization? *Sociology of Health and Illness.* 25, 7: 815–37.

Hislop J. and Arber, S. (2004) Understanding women's sleep management: beyond medicalization-healthicization: A response to Simon Williams. *Sociology of Health and Illness.* 26, 4: 460–3.

Hobbes, T. (1985/1651) *Leviathan* (with an introduction by J.B. McPherson). London: Penguin.

Hobson, A. (1995) *Sleep.* New York: Scientific American Library.

Hobson, A. (2002) *Dreaming: An Introduction to the Science of Sleep.* Oxford: Oxford University Press.

Hochschild, A.R. (1983) *The Managed Heart: The Commercialization of Human Feeling.* Berkeley CA: University of California Press.

Hochschild, A.R. (1994) The commercial spirit of intimate life and the abduction of feminism: signs from women's advice books. *Theory, Culture and Society.* 11: 1–24.

Hochschild, A.R. (1997) *The Time Bind: When Work Becomes Home and Home Becomes Work.* New York: Metropolitan Press.

Hochschild, A.R. with A. Machung (1990) *The Second Shift: Working Parents and the Revolution at Home.* London: Piatkus.

Holdbrook, A.M. (2004) Treating insomnia: use of drugs is rising despite evidence of harm and little meaningful benefit. *British Medical Journal.* 329, 20th November: 1198–9.

Hollyer, B. and Smith, L. (2002) *Sleep: The Easy Way to Peaceful Nights.* London: Cassell.

Honoré, C. (2004) *In Praise of Slowness: How a World Wide Movement is Challenging the Cult of Speed.* London: Orion Books.

Horne, J. (1999) Vehicle accidents related to sleep. *Occupational Environmental Medicine.* 56: 289–94.

Hume, K.I., Van, F. and Watson, A. (1998) A field study of age and gender differences in habitual adult sleep. *Journal of Sleep Research.* 7: 85–94.

Hunter, A. (1808) *Men and Manners.* London: Chapman and Hall.

Huntley, R. (1997) *The Sleep Book for Tired Parents.* London: Souvenir.

Hyppä, M.T. and Kronholm, E. (1987) How does Finland sleep? *Social Insurance Institution ML 68,* Turku, Finland.

Hyppä, M., Kronholm, E. and Alanen, E. (1997) Quality of sleep during economic recession in Finland: a longitudinal cohort study. *Social Science and Medicine*. 45, 5: 731–8.

Idzikowski, C. (1999) *The Insomnia Kit*. Dublin: Newleaf.

Idzikowski, C. (2000) *Learn to Sleep Well: Proven Strategies for Getting to Sleep and Staying Asleep*. London: Duncan Baird Publications.

Illich, I. (1975) *Medicial Nemesis*. London: Calder and Boyars.

Institute of Medicine (1979) *Sleeping Pills, Insomnia and Medical Practice*. Washington DC: National Academy of Sciences.

Jacobson, E. (1938) *You Can Sleep Well: The ABCs of Restful Sleep for the Average Person*. New York/London: Whittlesey House.

Johns, M.W. (1991) A new method for measuring daytime sleepiness: the Epworth Sleepiness Scale. *Sleep*. 14: 540–5.

Johns, M.W. and Hocking, B. (1997) Daytime sleepiness and sleep habits of Australian workers. *Sleep*. 20, 10: 844–9.

Johnson, S. (2003/1739–61) *Samuel Johnson: Selected Essays* (with an introduction by D. Womersley). London: Penguin.

Jouvet, M. (1965) Paradoxical sleep: a study of its nature and its mechanism. *Progress in Brain Research*. 18: 20–57.

Jouvet, M. (1999) *The Paradox of Sleep: The Story of Dreaming* (translated by L. Garey). Cambridge MA: MIT Press.

Jouvet, M. and Mounier, D. (1960) Effects des lesions de la formation reticular pontique sur le sommeil du chat. *Comptes Rendus des Seances de la Société de Biologie et de ses Filiales*. 154: 2301–5.

Jouvet, M., Michel, F and Courjon, J. (1959) Sur un stade d'activite electrique cerebrale rapide au cours du sommeil physiologique. *Comptes Rendus des Seances de la Société de Biologie et de ses Filiales*. 153: 1024–8.

Kales, A. (1969) *Sleep: Physiology and Pathology*. Philadelphia PA: Lippincott.

Kales, A. and Kales, J.D. (1970) Sleep laboratory and evaluation of psychoactive drugs. *Pharmacology for Physicians*. 4: 1–6.

Kales, A., Malmstrom, E.J. and Scharf, M.B. (1969) Psychophysiological and biochemical changes following use and withdrawal of hypnotics, in A. Kales (ed.) *Sleep: Physiology and Pathology*. Philadelphia PA: J.P. Lippincott.

Karasek, R. and Theorell, T. (1990) *Healthy Work: Stress, Productivity, and the Reconstruction of Working Life*. New York: Basic Books.

Kiley, J.P. (2000) Foreword, in M.H. Kryger, T. Roth and W.C. Dement (eds) *Principles and Practice of Sleep Medicine* (3rd edn). Philadelphia/London: W.B. Saunders.

Kirwan-Taylor, H. (2001) Snooze control. *The Sunday Times*. (Style Supplement), 13th May: 31.

Kleitman, N. (1927) Studies on the physiology of sleep: v. some experiments on puppies. *American Journal of Physiology*. 84: 386–95.

Kleitman, N. (1963/1939) *Sleep and Wakefulness* (revised and enlarged edition). Chicago IL/London: University of Chicago Press.

Kress, N. (1993) *Beggars in Spain*. New York: EOS/Harper Collins.

Kress, N. (1995) *Beggars and Choosers*. New York: Tor.

Kress, N. (1996) *Beggars Ride*. New York: Tor.

Kripke, D.F., Simons, R.N., Garfinkel, L. and Hammond, E.C. (1979) Short and long sleep and sleeping pills: is increased mortality associated? *Archives of General Psychiatry*. 36: 103–16.

Kroker, K. (2005) *The Sleep of Others*. Toronto: University of Toronto Press.

Kroll-Smith, S. (2000) The social production of the drowsy person. *Perspectives on Social Problems*. 12: 89–109.

Kroll-Smith, S. (2003) Popular media and 'excessive daytime sleepiness': a study of rhetorical authority in medical sociology. *Sociology of Health and Illness*. 25, 6: 625–43.

Kryger, M.H. (1983) Sleep apnea: from the needles of Dionysius to continuous positive airway pressure. *Archives of Internal Medicine*. 143: 2301–8.

Kryger, M.H. (1995) Is society sleep deprived? *Sleep*. 18, 10: 901.

Kryger, M.H., Roth, T. and Dement, W.C. (eds) (2000a) *Principles and Practice of Sleep Medicine* (3rd edn). Philadelphia/London: W.B. Saunders.

Kryger, M.H., Roth, T. and Dement, W.C. (eds) (2000b) Editors' Preface, in M.H. Kryger, T. Roth and W.C. Dement, *Principles and Practice of Sleep Medicine* (3rd edn). Philadelphia/London: W.B. Saunders.

Kryger, M.H., Roth, T. and Dement, W.C. (eds) (2005) *Principles and Practice of Sleep Medicine* (4th edn). Philadelphia/London: W.B. Saunders.

La Berge, S. (1980) Lucid dreaming as a learnable skill: a case study. *Perceptual and Motor Skills*. 51: 1039–42.

La Berge, S. (1985) *Lucid Dreaming*. Los Angeles CA: JP Tarcher.

La Berge, S. and Dement, W.C. (1982) Voluntary control of respiration during REM sleep. *Sleep Research*. 11: 107.

La Berge, S. and Rheingold, H. (1990) *Exploring the World of Lucid Dreaming*. New York: Ballantine Books.

La Berge, S., Nagel, L., Dement, W.C. and Zarcone, V. Jnr (1981) Lucid dreaming verified by volitional communication during REM sleep. *Perceptual and Motor Skills*. 52: 727–32.

Lavie, P. (1986) Nothing new under the moon: historical accounts of sleep apnea syndrome. *Archives of Internal Medicine*. 144: 2025–8.

Lawton, J. (2000) *The Dying Process: Patients' Experience of Palliative Care*. London: Routledge.

Lazarus, R. and Folkman, S. (1984) *Stress, Appraisal and Coping*. New York: Springer.

Leadbeater, C. (2004) *Dream On: Sleep in the 24/7 Society*. London: Demos.

Leadbeater, C. and Wilsdon J. (2003) Time for bed. *Green Futures*. November/December: 40–2.

Leder, D. (1990) *The Absent Body*. Chicago IL: University of Chicago Press.

Lee-Treweek, G. (2001) Bedroom abuse: the hidden work in a nursing home, in M. Allott and M. Robb (eds) *Understanding Health and Social Care: An Introductory Reader*. London: Sage Publications.

Legendre, R. (1912) De la propriété hypnotoxique de humeurs developpée au cours d'une veille prolongée. *Comptes Rendus des Seances de la Société de Biologie et de ses Filiales*. 72: 210–12.

Lemmey, D., McFarlane, J., Willson, P. and Maecha, A. (2001) Intimate partner violence: mothers' perspectives of effects on their children. *American Journal of Maternal Child Nursing*. 26, 2 (March–April): 98–103.

Levi, P. (1987/1958) *If This is a Man and The Truce* (translated by S. Wolf with an introduction by P. Bailey and an Afterword by the author). London: Abacus.

Levin, M. (1934) Narcolepsy in the Machine Age: the recent increase in the incidence of narcolepsy. *The Journal of Neurology and Psychopathology*. 15: 60–4.

Lewis, K.E., Blagrove, M. and Ebden, P. (2002) Sleep deprivation and junior doctors' performance. *Postgraduate Medical Journal*. 78: 85–7.

Li, Y. (2003) Discourse of mid-day napping: a political windsock in contemporary China, in B. Steger and L. Brunt (2003) *Night-time and Sleep in Asia and the West: Exploring the Dark Side of Life*. London: Routledge Curzon.

Loomis, A.L., Harvey, E.N. and Hobart, G.A. (1935a) Electrical potentials of the human brain. *Science*. 81: 1597–8.

Loomis, A.L., Harvey, E.N. and Hobart, G.A. (1935b) Further observations on the potential rhythms of the cerebral cortex during sleep. *Science*. 82: 198–200.

Lott, M.A. (1970) Editor's notes to *Hamlet: New Swan Shakespeare Advanced Series*. London: Longman.

Lowenberg, J. and Davis, F. (1994) Beyond medicalization-demedicalization: the case of holistic health. *Sociology of Health and Illness*. 16, 5: 579–99.

Lozoff, B. (1995) Culture and family: influences on childhood sleep practices and problems, in R. Ferber and M. Kryger (eds) *Principles and Practice of Sleep Medicine in the Child*. Philadelphia/London: W.B. Saunders.

Lupton, D. (1997) Foucault and the medicalisation critique, in A. Petersen and R. Bunton (eds) *Foucault, Health and Medicine*. London: Routledge.

Lupton, D. and Barclay, L. (1997) *Constructing Fatherhood: Discourses and Experiences*. London: Sage Publications.

MacNish, R. (1859) *The Philosophy of Sleep* (revised edition). Glasgow/London: M.R. M'Phun.

Malcolm, N. (1959) *Dreaming*. London: Routledge and Kegan Paul.

Marcus, C.L. and Loughlin, G.M. (1996) Effect of sleep deprivation on driving safety in house staff. *Sleep*. 19: 763.

Marmot, M. and Wilkinson, R. (eds) (1999) *Social Determinants of Health*. Oxford: Oxford University Press.

Marquez, G.G. (1970/1967) *One Hundred Years of Solitude* (translated by G. Rabassa). London: Jonathan Cape.

Martin, E. (1987) *The Woman in the Body*. Buckingham: Open University Press.

Martin, E. (1994) *Flexible Bodies: The Role of Immunology in American Culture from the Age of Polio to the Age of AIDS*. Boston MA: Beacon Press.

Martin, E. (2000) Flexible bodies: science and a new culture of health in the US, in S. Williams, J. Gabe and M. Calnan (eds) *Health, Medicine and Society: Key Theories, Future Agendas*. London: Routledge.

Martin, P. (2003) *Counting Sheep: The Science and Pleasures of Sleep and Dreams*. London: Flamingo.

Mattiason, I., Lingärde, F., Nilsson, J.A. and Theorell, T. (1990) Threat of unemployment and cardiovascular risk factors: longitudinal study of quality of sleep and serum cholesterol concentrations in men threatened with redundancy. *British Medical Journal*. 301: 461–6.

Mauss, M. (1973/1934) Techniques of the body. *Economy and Society*. 2: 70–88.

Mavromatis, A. (1987) *Hypnagogia: The Unique State of Consciousness Between Wakefulness and Sleep*. London: Routledge.

Mayall, B. (1996) *Children, Health and the Social Order*. Buckingham: Open University Press.

Mayall, B. (2002) *Towards a Sociology for Childhood*. Buckingham: Open University Press.

Mayhew, H. (nd.) *Mayhew's London, Being Selected from 'London Labour and the London Poor' (first published in 1851)*. London: Spring Books.

Melbin, M. (1978) Night as frontier. *American Sociological Review*. 43, 1: 3–22.

Melbin, M. (1989) *Night as Frontier: Colonizing the World after Dark*. London: Macmillan.

Melechi, A. (2003) *Fugitive Minds: On Madness, Sleep and other Twilight Affections*. London: William Heinemann.

Mennell, S. (1989) *Norbert Elias: Civilization and the Human Self-image*. Oxford: Blackwell.

Merleau-Ponty, M. (1962) *The Phenomenology of Perception*. London: Routledge.

Mertin, P. and Mohr, P.B. (2002) Incidence and correlates of posttrauma symptoms in children from backgrounds of domestic violence. *Violence and Victims*. 17, 5 (October): 555–67.

Mitler, M.M., Dement, W.C. and Dinges, D.F. (2000) Sleep medicine, public policy, and public health, in M.H. Kryger, T. Roth and W.C. Dement (eds) *Principles and Practice of Sleep Medicine* (3rd edn). Philadelphia/London: W.B. Saunders.

Mizen, P., Bolton, A. and Pole, C. (1999) School age workers: the paid employment of children in Britain. *Work, Employment and Society*. 13, 3: 423–38.

Mizen, P., Pole, C. and Bolton, A. (eds) (2001) *Hidden Hands: International Perspectives on Children's Work and Labour*. London: RoutledgeFalmer.

Moore-Ede, M. (1993) *The 24 Society: The Risks, Costs and Consequences of a World That Never Stops*. London: Piatkus.

Morgan, K. (1987) *Sleep and Ageing*. London/Sydney: Croom Helm.

Morgan, K., Dixon, S., Mathers, N., Thompson, J. and Tomeny, M. (2004) Psychological treatment for insomnia in the regulation of long-term hypnotic drug use. *Health Technology Assessment*. 8, 8: 1–80.

Moruzzi, G. and Magoun, H.W. (1949) Brain stem reticular formation and activation of the EEG. *Electroencephalography and Clinical Neurophysiology*. 1: 455–73.

Murdoch, I. (1973) *The Black Prince*. London: Chatto and Windus.

National Commission on Sleep Disorders Research (1993) *Wake Up America: A National Sleep Alert. V. 1: Executive Summary and Executive Report of the NCSDR*. Washington DC: NCSDR.

Netzer, N.C. (2002) Sleep medicine before and after Dickens. *Sleep and Breathing*. 6, Part 1: 41–4.

Newton, T. with J. Handy and S. Fineman (1995) *'Managing' Stress: Emotion and Power at Work*. London: Sage Publications.

Norbutt, M. (2004) Waking up to sleep clinics: growing industry offers eye-catching investments. *American Medical Association News*, 5th January (www.ama-assn.org/amednews/2004/01/05/bisa015.htm).

NSF (National Sleep Foundation) (1997) *Gallup Survey: Sleepiness in America* (www.sleepfoundation.org/publications/SleepinessInAmerica.cfm).

NSF (2000) *Survey of Primary Care Physicians*. (www.sleepfoundation.org).

NSF (2001) *2001: Sleep in America Poll* (www.sleepfoundation.org).

NSF (2002) *2002: Sleep in America Poll* (www.sleepfoundation.org).

NSF (2003) *2003: Sleep in America Poll* (www.sleepfoundation.org).

NSF (2004) *2004: Sleep in America Poll* (www.sleepfoundation.org).

NSF (nd) The importance of sleep (www.sleepfoundation.org/about.cfm).

O'Dea, W. (1958) *The Social History of Lighting*. London: Hamish Hamilton.

Oakley, A. (1984) *The Captured Womb*. Oxford: Blackwell.

Office of the Deputy Prime Minister (1999) *Coming in From the Cold: The Government's Strategy on Rough Sleeping*. London: ODPM.

Ohida, T., Kamal, A.M.M., Uchiyama, M., Kim, K., Takemura, S., Sone, T. and Ishii, T. (2001) The influence of lifestyle and health status on sleep loss among the Japanese population. *Sleep*. 24, 3: 333–7.

Onion, A. (2003) The no-doze soldier: military seeking radical ways of stumping need for sleep (http://abcnews.go.com/sections/scitech/DailyNews/nosleep021218.html).

ONS (Office for National Statistics) (2003) Summary results: What we do, when and with whom. UK 2000 Time Use Survey (www.statistics.gov.uk/timeuse/summary_results).

Orwell, G. (2003/1933) *Down and Out in Paris and London*. London: Penguin.

Oswald, I. (1968) Drugs and sleep. *Pharmacological Review*. 20: 272–303.

Oswald, I. and Priest, R. (1965) Five weeks to escape the sleeping pill habit. *British Medical Journal*. 2: 1093–5.

Owens, J.L., France, K.G. and Wiggs, L. (1999) Behavioural and cognitive-behavioural interventions for sleep disorders in infants and children: a review. *Sleep Medicine Reviews*. 3: 281–302.

Pantley, E. (2002) *The No-cry Sleep Solution: Gentle Ways to Help Your Baby Sleep Through the Night*. Chicago/London: Contemporary Books.

Parsons, T. (1951) *The Social System*. London: Routledge and Kegan Paul.

Partinen, M. and Hublin, C. (2000) Epidemiology of sleep disorders, in M.H. Kryger, T. Roth and W.C. Dement (eds) *Principles and Practice of Sleep Medicine* (3rd edn). Philadelphia/London: W.B. Saunders.

Partinen, M., Eskelinen, L. and Tuomi, K. (1984) Complaints of insomnia in different occupations. *Scandinavian Journal of Work and Environmental Health*. 10 (6: Special No.): 467–9.

Passouant, P. (1981) Doctor Gelineau (1826–1906): narcolepsy centennial. *Sleep*. 3: 241–6.

Patton, D.V., Landers, D.R. and Agarwall, I.T. (2001) Sleep deprivation among resident physicians. *Journal of Health Law*. 34, 3 (Summer): 377–417.

Pavlov, I.P. (1923) The identity of inhibition with sleep and hypnosis. *Science Monthly*. 17: 603–8.

Pavlov, I.P. (1927) *Conditioned Reflexes: An Investigation of the Physiological Activity of the Cerebral Cortext*. New York: Oxford University Press.

Pavlov, I.P. (1928) *Lectures on Conditioned Reflexes*. London: Lawrence and Wishart.

Pearce, J. and Bidder, J. (1999) *The New Baby and Toddler Sleep Programme: How to Have a Peaceful Night* (new edition). London: Vermillion.

Pepys, S. (1993/1660–69) *The Shorter Pepys* (selected and edited by R. Latham). London: Penguin.

Phelan, M., Akram, G., Lewis, M., Blenkinsopp, A., Millson, D. and Croft, P.

(2002) A community-pharmacy-based survey of users of over-the-counter sleep aids. *The Pharmaceutical Journal.* 269, 31 August: 287–90.

Phillipson, E.A. (1993) Sleep apnoea – a major public health problem. *New England Journal of Medicine.* 328: 1271–3.

Pick, D. and Roper, L. (2004) Introduction. In D. Pick and L. Roper (eds) *Dreams and History: The Interpretation of Dreams from Ancient Greece to Modern Psychoanalysis.* London/NY: Brunner-Routledge.

Pickersgill, T. (2001) The European Working Time Directive for doctors in training. *British Medical Journal.* 323: 1266.

Pieron, H. (1913) *Le Probleme Physiologique du Sommeil.* Paris: Masson et Cie.

Popay, J. (1990) 'My health is alright, but I'm just tired all the time', in H. Roberts (ed.) *Women's Health Matters.* London: Routledge.

Proust, M. (2002) *In Search of Lost Time [A la recherché du temps perdu].* (translated by C.K. Scott Moncrieff and T. Kilmartin, revised by D.J. Enright). London: Vintage.

Radice, S. (2003) The night shift: can couples who sleep apart really stay together. *The Guardian.* 9th May: 7.

Rechtschaffen, A. and Kales, A. (1968) *A Manual of Standardized Terminology, Techniques and Scoring System for Sleep Stages of Human Subjects.* Bethesda: US Dept. of Health, Education and Welfare, Public Health Service.

Rechtschaffen, A., Bergman, B.M., Everson, C.A., Kushida, C.A. and Gilliland, M.A. (1989) Sleep deprivation in the rat: X. integration and discussion of the findings. *Sleep.* 12: 68–87.

Reeves, R. (2003) The precious time poll: about time. *The Observer.* (Real Time, special supplement) 29 June.

Reidiech, M., Reis, J. and Creason, M. (1990) Sleep in old age: focus on gender differences. *Sleep.* 13, 5: 410–24.

Reisman, C.K. (1989) Women and medicalization: a new perspective, in P. Brown (ed.) *Perspectives in Medical Sociology.* Belmont CA: Wadsworth Publishing.

Rensen, P. (2003) Sleeping without a home: the embedment of sleep in the lives of the rough-sleeping homeless in Amsterdam, in B. Steger and L. Brunt (2003) *Night-time and Sleep in Asia and the West: Exploring the Dark Side of Life.* London: Routledge Curzon.

Richardson, G.S., Wyatt, J.K., Sullivan, J.P., Orav, E.J., Ward, A.E., Wolf, M.A. and Czeisler, C.A. (1996) Objective assessment of sleep and alertness in medical house staff and the impact of protected time for sleep. *Sleep.* 19, 9: 718–26.

Richter, A. (2003) Sleeping time in early Chinese literature, in B. Steger and L. Brunt (2003) *Night-time and Sleep in Asia and the West: Exploring the Dark Side of Life.* London: Routledge Curzon.

Russell, B. (2004/1933) *In Praise of Idleness* (with a preface by A. Gottlieb, and introduction by H. Woodshouse). London: Routledge.

Sacks, O. (1990/1973) *Awakenings.* London: Picador.

Sadeh, V. (2001) *Sleeping Like a Baby: A Sensitive Approach to Solving Your Child's Sleep Problems.* New Haven/London: Yale University Press.

Sample, I. (2005) Sleeping around the horn. *The Guardian.* 12th February: 9.

Sample, I. and Evans, R. (2004) MoD bought thousands of stay awake pills in advance of the war on Iraq. *The Guardian.* 29th July: 1.

Sanofi-Synthelabo, Inc. (2004) Very robust growth in developed sales in 2003. January 2004 (www.sanofi-synthelabo.us).

Sartre, J.-P. (2001/1939) *Sketch for a Theory of the Emotions*. London: Routledge.

Scambler, G. (1989) *Epilepsy*. London: Routledge.

Schutz, A. with T. Luckman (1974/1973) *The Structures of the Lifeworld* (translated by R.M. Zaner and H.T. Englehardt Jnr). London: Heinemann.

Schwartz, B. (1970) Notes on the sociology of sleep. *Sociological Quarterly*. 11: 485–99.

Scott, A. (2004) Sleep tight: Britain's first taste of the Japanese short-stay capsule hotel will pack a lot of luxury into a little space. *The Guardian*. 13th September: 5.

Sennett, R. (1998) *The Corrosion of Character: The Personal Consequences of Work in the New Capitalism*. London: W.W. Norton & Co.

Serge, V. (1970) *Men in Prison*. London: Gollancz.

Shamadsani, S. (2003) *Jung and the Making of Modern Psychology: the Dream of Science*. Cambridge: Cambridge University Press.

Shapiro, C.M. (ed.) (1994) *The ABC of Sleep Disorders*. London: BMJ Publications.

Shapiro, C.M., Caterrall, J.R., Oswald, I. and Flenley, D.C. (1981) Where are the British sleep apnoea patients? *Lancet*. 2: 523.

Showalter, E. (1997) *Hystories: Hysterical Epidemics and Modern Culture*. London: Picador.

Siegrist, J., Peter, R., Junge, A., Cremer, P., Seidel, D. (1990) Low status control, high effort at work and ischaemic heart disease: prospective evidence from blue-collar men. *Social Science and Medicine*. 31: 1127–1134.

Sleep Council (2002) *Separate Beds – The Secret of Wedded Bliss* (www.sleepcouncil.com).

Smith, R.J. (1979) Study finds sleeping pills overprescribed. *Science*. 204: 287–8.

Solzhenitsyn, A. (1968) *One Day in the Life of Ivan Denisovich*. Harmondsworth: Penguin.

Souter, R.L. and Wilson, J.A. (1986) Does hospital noise disturb patients? *British Medical Journal*. 292: 305.

Speaker, S.L. (1997) From 'happiness pills' to 'national nightmare': changing cultural assessment of minor tranquilizers in America 1955–1980. *Journal of the History of Medicine*. 52: 338–76.

Spradley, J.A. (1970) *You Owe Yourself a Drink: An Ethnography of Urban Nomads*. Boston MA: Little, Brown.

Stacey, M. (1988) *The Sociology of Health and Healing*. London: Routledge.

Stampi, C. (1992) *Why We Nap: Evolution, Chronobiology and the Functions of Polyphasic and Ultrashort Sleep*. Basel: Birkhauser Verlag

Stanley, N. (2004) Personal communication. June.

Steger, B. (2003a) Negotiating sleep patterns in Japan, in B. Steger and L. Brunt (2003) *Night-time and Sleep in Asia and the West: Exploring the Dark Side of Life*. London: Routledge Curzon.

Steger, B. (2003b) Getting *away* with sleep – social and cultural aspects of dozing in parliament. *Social Science Japan Journal*. 6: 181–97.

Steger, B. and Brunt, L. (eds) (2003) *Night-time and Sleep in Asia and the West: Exploring the Dark Side of Life*. London: Routledge Curzon.

Stoker, B. (1993/1897) *Dracula*. London: Penguin.

Stopes, M.C. (1918) *Married Love*. London: G.P. Putnam's Sons.

Stopes, M.C. (1956) *Sleep*. London: Chatto and Windus.

Stores, G. and Crawford, C. (1998) Medical student education in sleep and its disorders. *Journal of the Royal College of Physicians of London*. 32, 2: 149–53.

Stradling, J.R. and Davies, R.J.O. (1997) Obstructive sleep apnoea: evidence for efficacy of continuous positive airways pressure is compelling. *British Medical Journal*. 315: 368.

Strong, P. (1979) Sociological imperialism and the medical profession: a critical examination of the thesis of medical imperialism. *Social Science and Medicine*. 13A: 199–216.

Taft, A., Broom, D.H. and Legge, D. (2004) General practitioner management of intimate partner abuse and the whole family: qualitative study. *British Medical Journal*, doi:10.1136/bmj.38014.626535.OB (published 6 February): 1–4.

Tart, C. (1988) From spontaneous event to lucidity: a review of attempts to consciously control nocturnal dreaming, in J. Gackenbach and S. La Berge (eds.) *Conscious Mind, Dreaming Brain*. New York: Plenum Press.

Taylor, B. (1993) Unconsciousness and society: the sociology of sleep. *International Journal of Politics and Culture*. 6: 463–71.

Taylor, N. (2003) What's it worth? The value of our hours across the globe. *The Observer (Real Time Supplement)*, 29th June.

Thompson, E.P. (1967) Time, work discipline and industrial capitalism. *Past and Present*. 38 (December): 56–97.

Thorpy, M. (1991) History of sleep and man, in M. Thorpy and J. Yager (eds.) *The Encyclopaedia of Sleep and Sleep Disorders*, New York: Facts on File.

Thorpy, M. (2000) Classification of sleep disorders, in M.H. Kryger, T. Roth and W.C. Dement (eds) *Principles and Practice of Sleep Medicine* (3rd edn). Philadelphia/London: W.B. Saunders.

Thorpy, M. and Yager, J. (eds.) (1991) *The Encyclopaedia of Sleep and Sleep Disorders*, New York: Facts on File.

Townsend, P. (1962) *The Last Refuge*. London: Routledge and Kegan Paul.

TUC (Trades Union Congress) (2002) *About Time: A New Agenda for Shaping Working Hours*. London: TUC.

Turner, B.S. (1992) *Max Weber: From History to Modernity*. London: Routledge.

Valagin, Francis de (1768) *A Treatise on Diet, or the Management of Human Life*. London: J.W. Oliver.

Van den Bulck, J. (2003) Text messaging as a cause of sleep interruption in adolescents, evidence from a cross-sectional study. *Journal of Sleep Research*. 12, 3 (Sep): 263.

Van den Bulck, J. (2004) Television viewing, computer game playing, and Internet use and self-reported time to bed and time out of bed in secondary-school children. *Sleep*. 27, pt. 1 (Feb): 101–4.

Van Der Zee, B. (1997) *The New Green Pharmacy: The Story of Western Herbal Medicine*. London: Vermillion.

van Eeden, F. (1913) A study of dreams. *Proceedings of the Society for Psychical Research*. 26: 431–45.

Van Straten, M. (1996) *The Good Sleep Guide*. London: Kyle Cathie.

Virilio, P. (1986) *Speed and Politics: An Essay on Dromology*, transl. M. Polizotti. New York: Semiotext(e).

von Economo, C. (1928) Theorie du sommeil. *Journal of Neurological Psychiatry* 28: 437–64.

von Economo, C. (1930) Sleep as a problem of localisation. *Journal of Nervous Mental Disease*. 71: 249–59.

von Economo, C. (1931) *Encephalitis Lethargica: Its Sequelae and Treatment*. Oxford: Oxford University Press.

von Schubert, G.H. (1968/1814) *Die Symbolik des Traumes*. Stuttgart: Besler Presse.

Wadd, W. (1822/1816) *Cursory Remarks on Corpulence; or Obesity Considered as a Disease: With a Critical Examination of Ancient and Modern Opinions Relative to its Causes and Cure* (3rd edn). London: Gallow Medical Bookseller.

Wainwright, D. and Calnan, M. (2002) *Work Stress: The Making of a Modern Epidemic*. Buckingham: Open University Press.

Wainwright, M. (2002) Dozing driver who caused 10 deaths gets five years. *The Guardian*. 12 January: 1.

Walter Reid Army Institute of Research (1997) *Sleep, Sleep Deprivation and Human Performance*. Bethesda MD: WRAIR, Dept. of Behavioral Biology (www.wrair.army.mil/depts/behavbio).

Watson, J. (2000) *Male Bodies: Health, Culture and Identity*. Buckingham: Open University Press.

Webb, W.B. (1975) *Sleep: The Gentle Tyrant*. Englewood Cliffs, NJ: Prentice Hall.

Webb, W.B. and Agnew, H.W. (1975) Are we chronically sleep deprived? *Bulletin of the Psychonomic Society*. 6: 47–8.

Weber, M. (1974/1930) *The Protestant Ethic and the Spirit of Capitalism*. (translated by T. Parsons, foreword by R. Tawney) London: Unwin University Books.

Weir Mitchell, S. (1890) Some disorders of sleep. *American Journal of the Medical Sciences*. 100: 109–27.

Welford, H. (1999) *Helping your Baby or Child to Sleep*. London: Marshall.

Welsh, E., Buchanan, A., Flouri, E. and Lewis, J. (2004) *'Involved' Fathering and Child Well-being*. London: National Children's Bureau (for the Joseph Rowntree Foundation).

WHO (World Health Organization) (2004) *Technical Meeting on Sleep and Health*. European Centre for Environment and Health, Bonn office, Germany (www.euro.who.int/noise/activities).

Wiggs, L. (2004) *Children and Sleep (a Report commissioned for Horlick)*. Oxford: University of Oxford, Department of Psychiarty.

Wilkoff, W.G. (2000) *Is My Child Overtired?: The Sleep Solution for Raising Happier, Healthier Children*. New York/London: Simon and Schuster.

Williams, S.J. (2001) Sociological imperialism and the medical profession: Where are we now? *Sociology of Health and Illness*. 23: 135–58.

Williams, S.J. (2004) Beyond medicalization-healthicization? A rejoinder to Hislop and Arber. *Sociology of Health and Illness*. 26, 4: 453–9.

Williams, S.J. and Boden, S. (2004) Consumed with sleep? Dormant bodies in consumer culture. *Sociological Research Online*. 9, 2 www.socresonline.org.uk/9/2/willliams.html.

Williams S.J. and Calnan, M. (eds.) (1996) *Modern Medicine: Lay Perspectives and Experiences*. London: UCL Press.

Williams, S.J., Griffiths, F.E. and Lowe, P. (2004) *Sleep: A Feasibility Study*. University of Warwick.

Williams, S.J., Humphreys, C. and Lowe, P. (2004) *Sleep and Domestic Violence: A Pilot Study*. University of Warwick.

Willis, T. (1692) *The London Practice of Physick*. London: Thomas Basset.

Wilson, H. (2004) Sleep your way to the top. *The Guardian*. 16th February (Office Hours): 5.

Wingard, D.L. and Berkman, L.F. (1983) Mortality risk associated with sleeping patterns among adults. *Sleep*. 6, 2: 102–7.

Winterman, D. (2004) Sleeping on the job. *BBC News Online Magazine*, 7th September. http://news.bbc.co.uk/1/hi/magazine/3631040.stm.

Wohl, A.S. (1976) Sex and the single room: incest among the Victorian working-classes, in A.S. Wohl (ed.) *The Victorian Family: Structure and Stresses*. London: Croom Helm.

Wouters, C. (1986) Formalization and informalization: changing tension balances in civilizing processes. *Theory, Culture and Society*. 3, 2: 1–18.

Wouters, C. (1987) Developments in the behavioural codes between the sexes: the formalization of informalization in The Netherlands 1930–85. *Theory, Culture and Society*. 4(2–3): 405–27.

Wright, J., Johns, R., Watt, I., Melvitla, A. and Sheldon, T. (1997a) Health effects of obstructive sleep apnoea and the effectiveness of continuous positive airways pressure: systematic review of the research evidence. *British Medical Journal*. 314: 851–60, (plus Editorial 'Deep and shallow').

Wright, J., Johns, R., Watt, I., Melvitla, A. and Sheldon, T. (1997b) Obstructive sleep apnoea: author's reply. *British Medical Journal*. 315: 551.

Wright, L. (1962) *Warm and Snug: A History of the Bed*. London: Routledge and Kegan Paul.

Zeilinski, J., Polakowska, M., Kurjata, P., Kupsc, W. and Zgierska, S. (1998) Excessive daytime somnolence in adult population of Warsaw. *Polish Archives of Medicine, Wewn*. 99: 407–13

Zola, I.K. (1972) Medicine as an institution of social control. *Sociological Review*. 20: 487–503.

Index

24/7 society 104–5, 113, 137
absence from self 70
acceleration thesis 106
accidents; due to sleepiness 105, 114; sleep
   apnoea a cause of 150
Åckerstadt, T. 115
active/passive sleep 13–14, 15
ADHD (Attention Deficit/Hyperactivity
   Disorder) 151
Adler, A. 29
Africa, sleeping practices 108
age, and sleep 77–8, 89–90; daytime
   sleepiness 102; sleeping hours 139n
air 54–5
Alcmaeon 9–10
alternative therapies 21, 151, 161
Alvarez, A. 62, 63, 64
Ambien 151, 161
American Academy of Sleep Medicine 149
American Narcolepsy Association 147
American National Sleep Foundation 152
American Sleep Disorders Association 147
Amnesty International 135
Amsterdam, sleeping rough in 132–3
ancient Greeks 47; 'art of living' 47; beds of
   58; thought on sleep 9–10
animals, sleep of 34
Anthony, C. 118
Anthony, W.A. 118
anti-depressants 151
anxiolytics, prescriptions for 146
Arber, S. 86, 87, 92, 93, 95, 157–8
Archer, Jeffrey 127–8
Aristotle 10, 27, 32
Artemidorous 27, 28, 47
Asclepius, oracle of 27
Aserinsky, E. 16, 35n
Association for the Psychophysiological
   Study of Sleep 148
Association of Professional Sleep Societies 148
astronauts, beds of 61
atomism 10
Attention Deficit/Hyperactivity Disorder 151
Aubert, V. 2
Augustine 32
Australia, daytime sleepiness in 102

Ayukawa, J. 83

Ballard, J.G. 160
barbiturates 26, 151
Barker, Lady 56
Baxter, Richard 50
Baxter, V. 120
'beauty sleep', products 162
Bechterev, Vladimir Michailovitch 14
bedbugs 59–60
bedding 59, 60; marketing 172–3
bedroom 109; behaviour in 39, 41; privacy
   of 39–40; work in nursing homes 130–1
beds (see also sharing beds): airing 60–1; in
   Bible 38; care of 60; comfort of 61–2;
   history of 57–60; marketing 162
behavioural theories 13
Belensky, Col. 121, 122
Ben-Ari, E. 122–3, 124–5
Benedict, R. 140n
benzodiazepines 26, 146, 151
bereavement 94–5
Berger, Johannes 15
Bible, sleep in 37–9
biological clock 18–19; effect of artificial
   light on 45, 46
biphasic sleep patterns 108, 109
Blaxter, M. 103
blood 10, 11, 14
boarding schools 123
body: docile 48, 49; dormant 4, 32; ecstatic-
   recessive 68–9, 96
Boots, 'Healthy Living' products 161–2
Borde, A. 42
Bouchard, Abel 14
brain 11, 13–14; and dreams 30–1; electrical
   activity of 13, 15; wave patterns 15
Brannen, J. 84, 85
breathing 25
Bremer, Frederick 15
British Sleep Alliance 153
British Sleep Foundation 152
British Sleep Society 153
British Thoracic Society 153
Brokaw, J. 134
bromide 26

Brown-Sequard, Charles 14
Brunt, L. 108, 109, 110
Bunyan, John 96
Bury, M. 90
Bush, George W. 120

Calnan, M. 115, 116, 117
capitalism 50–1
Caton, Richard 15
causes of sleep, theories of 9–13
celebrities 163
Chadwick, Edwin, *Report on the Sanitary Conditions of the Labouring Population of Great Britain* 52–3
chemical theories of sleep 10, 13, 14
children: effect of domestic violence on sleep 134–5; pre-sleep activities 81–2; sharing a bed with 91; sleep patterns 78–84; sleep problems and ADHD 151; social organisation of sleep in day-care centres 123–6; and work 79, 82
China, sleeping patterns 109, 110–11, 119
chronobiology 12, 18
Churchill, W.S. 62, 120
Cicero 62
circadian cycle 18
civilization 39–47
Claparede, Édouard 14
Clarke, A. 165n
class 75; beds and 59–60; and sleep 42, 43, 44
CLOCK gene 98n
Coe, Jonathan 163
cognitive behavioural therapy 151
Cohen, S. 126
Coleridge, S.T. 22–3, 31, 96
commercialization of sleep 160–3
complete/incomplete sleep 13
concentration camps, sleep in 136
Confucianism 110
congestion theories of sleep 10, 13
Conrad, P. 144, 165n
continuous airways pressure (C-PAP) 147, 151, 153
controlling sleep 159–60
Coren, S. 105, 114
Cosnett, J. 24
couples, sleeping together 91–3, 95, 97
Crawford, C. 146
creativity, sleep and 46, 51
Crick, F. 36n
Crook, T. 52, 54, 55
Cropley, M. 115
Crossley, N. 75, 95, 170
cultures of sleep 108–11, 137

Dali, Salvador 31
darkness 63, 64
Davidson, H.C. 60
day-care centres, social organisation of children's sleep 123–6
daytime sleep (*see also* excessive daytime sleepiness; napping) 108–9, 109–10, 111, 150; in nursing homes 129–30

deafferentation theory 15, 16
death 95–6, 98
decision-making 79–80, 81
definition of sleep 33–4
Dekker, Thomas 65–6n
Dement, W.C. 13, 15, 16–17, 18–19, 102, 151, 152, 155
Dennett, D.C. 28
Descartes, René 11, 27, 28, 31
Diagnostic Classification of Sleep Disorders 147
Dickens, Charles 32; depiction of sleep disorders 23–4
digestion, sleep due to effects of 10
Dionysius 22
disappearance, phenomenology of 68–9, 96
disciples of Jesus, sleeping 38—9
disciplinary institutions 48–50, 55
divorce, and sleep patterns 95
doctors 145, 165n; lack of training in sleep disorders 146; and sleep clinics 150; working hours 114
Doi, Y. 140n
dolphins, sleep of 34
domestic violence 134–5
Donne, John 96
'dozing off' 129–30
dreams/dreaming 23, 27, 46, 68–9, 74; analysis of 47; Aristotle and 10; in Bible 38; creativity of 31; Freud and 28–31; history of 27–8; lucid 32–3, 34; manifest and latent content of 29, 31; REM sleep and 16, 18, 31, 32; time structure 72
duality of sleep 17, 18
Dubois, Raymond Emil 14
dyssomnias 166n

early adulthood, sleep patterns 84–5
'Easy Sleep' 118
Economo, Constantin von 14
Edison, Thomas 51
Eeden, Frederick van 31, 32
EEG (electroencephalograph) 13, 15, 17, 18
efficiency of sleep 117, 119, 140n
Egypt, beds in 58
Ekirch, R. 41–3, 44–6, 59
electric light, effect of on sleep 18, 45, 51, 63
Elias, N. 39, 40–1
Ellis, Havelock 32
Embodiment, sleep and 4–6, 67–100, 170, lifecourse and 77–90
Engels, F. 54
entertainment, consumption of sleep as 163
Epicurus 10
Erasmus 39
Europe, daytime sleepiness in 102
European Work Time Directive 114
excessive daytime sleepiness 102–3, 140n, 150, 152, 154; media and 154, 155
explanations for sleep, historic 9–16

falling asleep, phenomenology of 67–73

family, sleeping with 40, 41, 79
fears for safety 42, 44, 64, 134
financial hardship, effect on sleep 89
Finland, unemployment and sleep disruption 115–16
first/second sleep 45
Fitzgerald, M. 127
Flanagan, O. 29, 31
fleas 42, 44
flexible working 113
Flourens, Marie-Jean-Pierre 13
Ford, J. 23
Fordism 113, 119
Foster, M.A. 32
Foucault, M. 47—9
Fox, O. 32
Franklin, Benjamin 51
Freud, Sigmund 18, 32; *Interpretation of Dreams* 28–9, 30
functions of sleep 35, 36n

Galen 27
Galvini, Luigi 13
Gardner, Randy 20–1
Gelineau, Jean Baptiste 26
gender, and sleep (*see also* men; women) 78; daytime sleep 102
Geneva Conventions 135
Gleick, J. 106, 107
God, creation of seven-day week 37–8
Goffman, E. 75–6, 126
Golgi, Camillo 15
Greece, siesta 109
Green, C. 32
Green, W.E. 25
growing, during sleep 79
Gubrium, J.F. 129–30

Hall, W.W. 56
Haller, Albrecht von 12–13
hallucinations 20
hammocks 61
Hammond, W.A. 25
Harris, D.F. 57
Harrison, Y. 104
Hathaway, J.E. 134
Hayward, R. 29
health, sleep and 35, 56; shift work 113; sleep apnoea 150; sleepiness a risk to 102, 105, 114, 137–8; workplace 112, 114, 115–16
healthicisation 144, 154, 158–9
Hearne, K. 32
Heathrow, ruling by European Court of Human Rights 133–4
herbal remedies 21, 161
heroism, lack of sleep equated with 119
Hervey de Saint Deny, Leon 27, 32
Hess, W.R. 15
Hippocrates 10
Hislop, J. 86, 87, 92, 93, 95, 157–8
Hobbes, Thomas 27
Hobson, A. 19, 20, 30
Hochschild, A.R. 99n

Holstein, J.A. 129–30
homelessness 131–3
Honoré, C. 107
Horne, J. 104
hospitals 55; routine in 128; sleep in 128–9
hotels 123
hours of sleep 57, 102–3, 104; children 83; pre-industrial 42; social rank and 42; soldiers 121
housing 55
Hublin, C. 102, 115
human rights, sleep and 133–6, 138
Hunter, Alexander 26
hygiene of sleep 55–7
hypnagogic states 31, 46, 51, 70
hypnopompic states 31
Hypnos 47, 96
hypnotics 21, 25, 26, 161; prescriptions for 146, 151
hypnotoxin theory 14, 16

Imidazopyridines 151
imperialism, medicalisation and 144
inappropriate sleep 75
incest 52
inconsiderate sleepers 93
India, sleeping patterns 109
inemuri 76, 109, 110, 120, 126
inhibitory theories of sleep 14
insomnia 21, 24, 25; stress and 115
instinct, sleep as 14
interactional membrane 76–7
interactionism 5
inter-disciplinary research 171–2
Internet, sleep-related websites 155
Interpretation of Dreams (Freud) 28–9, 30
intervals of sleep 45–6
Iraq, torture of prisoners 135

Jacobson, Edmund 151
Japan: children's sleep in day-care centres 124–6; hours of sleep 103; nighttime youth culture 83; sleeping patterns 109, 111, 120
Johnson, Samuel 65n, 66n, 73
Joseph, dreams of 38
Jouvet, Michel 18
Jung, C.G. 29

Kiley, J.P. 149
Kleitman, N. 16–17, 26
Kress, N. 160
Kroll-Smith, S. 120, 154, 155–6
Kryger, M.H. 22

La Berge, S. 32–3
La Salle, J.B. 39—40
labour 50, 63
Ladies' Sanitary Association 56
larks and owls 78, 160
later life, sleep patterns 89–90
laudanum 43
Lavoisier, Antoine 54–5
lay/professional divide 155–6, 157

Leadbeater, C. 118
Leder, D. 68, 70, 71
Lee-Treweek, G. 130–1
Legalist philosophy 110
Legendre, Rene 14
legitimacy of sleep 75, 97
leisure, effect on sleep 106, 117
Leucippus 10
Levi, Primo 136
Li, Y. 111
Lifecourse, sleep and 77–90 (or see embodiment)
light see electric light
liminality of sleep 4–5, 70, 95–6
living conditions, Victorian 52–4
lodging shops/houses 53–4
Loomis, Alfred 15
Los Angeles, policing of rough sleepers 132
Louis XIV 60

MacArthur, Ellen 118–19
MacNish, Robert 13
magic, use of 43
Magoun, H.W. 15
main/side involvement 76, 109
Malcolm, N. 28, 32
Mann, Thomas 62
marketing 106, 160–3
Marquez, Gabriel Garcia 163
Martin, E 113, 143
Martin, P. 35n, 78, 115, 116, 121, 128, 135, 136
Martin, T.C. 51
Marx, Karl 63
masculinity 88–9, 98
Maupassant, Guy de 62
Maury, Alfred 31, 32
Mauss, M. 108
Mavromatis, A. 36n
Mayall, B. 80–1
measurement of sleepiness 139n
mechanistic explanation 11
media, role in medicalisation of sleep 154–6
medicalisation of sleep 5, 7, 143–54, 164–5; media and 154–6; resisting 156–9
medication 26–7, 130
medicine, sleep as 42
Melbin, M. 63–4, 159
Melechi, A. 32
men: as inconsiderate sleepers 93; quality of sleep 88; sleep patterns 88–9, 98; tiredness 85
Merleau-Ponty, M. 68, 69
mid-life, sleep patterns 86–9
MILD (mnemonic induction of lucid dreams) 32–3
military, study of sleep 121–2, 138, 159
Minowa, M. 140n
Mitchell, S.W. 25
Mitchison, G. 36n
Mitler, M.M. 103–4, 152
Modafinil 122, 159, 161
modernisation 111

Mohist philosophy 110
molecular genetics 160
Moliere 60
monasteries 48
monophasic sleep patterns 108–9
moods, sleep and 35
moral agendas 52, 54, 57
Morgan, K. 36n, 89
Moruzzi, G. 15
Moss, P. 84, 85
motherhood, sleep and 85–6, 86–7
Multiple Sleep Latency Test 139n
muscle atonia 18
Myers, Fredric 31, 32

napping 45, 76; children 124–5; in China 110–11; cluster 119; culture of 108, 109, 110; day beds for 60; Edison and 51; politicians' 120; power 107, 117, 118; soldiers 122; in workplace 117–20, 138
narcolepsy 26, 148, 152–3
Narcolepsy Association UK 152–3
NASA, 61
National Centre on Sleep Disorders Research 147
National Commission on Sleep Disorders Research 146
National Sleep Foundation 102, 146
negotiation of sleeping 5, 79–80, 97
neural theories of sleep 13
new management 113
Nietzsche, F. 32
nightmares 24, 134; magic used to divert 43
night-time: behaviour in 64–5; sleep in 109; social life in 63
nightwear 40, 42–3, 162
Norbutt, M. 149–50
normalisation of sleep problems 157
NREM sleep 17, 34, 78
nursing homes, sleep in 129–31
Nyx 96

obesity 22, 25, 150
occupation, effect on sleeping problems 112–13
opponent-process model 18–19
Ortous de Mairan, Jean Jacques d' 12, 18
Orwell, George 131
overcrowding 52
over-the-counter products 161
owls 78, 160

pain, and sleep disruption 43, 128
parasomnias 166n
parenting skills 151
Parsons, T. 73
Partinen, M. 102, 115
passive sleep 13–14, 15, 17
pathologies of sleep see sleep disorders
patient groups 152
patterns of sleep 77–8, 101; culture and 108–11; at work 112–20
Pavlov, Ivan P. 14